Feeding Herbs to Horses

Wendy & Terry Jennings

Published by Newlad Publishing Company

No part of this book may be reproduced or transmitted in any way or by any means, electronic or mechanical, including photocopy or any information storage and retrieval system, without permission in written form from the copyright holder.

All rights reserved.

Copyright Wendy and Terry Jennings 2000.

ISBN: 0 9538670-0-5.

Published June 2000.

Reprinted September 2000.

Published by Newlad Publishing Company

THE AUTHORS

Wendy and Terry Jennings have broad experience in caring for horses over many years. From the first family pony to running a thoroughbred stud near Newmarket, they have had direct personal involvement in the day to day care and management of countless horses. From their own competitive riding to preparing group winning racehorses, they have shared in the highs and lows which come with a dedication and love of the horse. Many night hours have been spent foaling mares or attending to the unwell horse, followed by full days of preparing youngsters for their future careers in the discipline best suited for their individual qualities. The joy of owning a winner at Royal Ascot is unique, but it cannot remove the sadness of losing a favourite horse. Wendy and Terry Jennings have had most of the ups and downs with horses that we dream of and dread.

Wendy Jennings special expertise in preparing herbal formulations started long before her involvement in the family owned stud, but it was during those years that she developed her knowledge and understanding of the wide ranging benefits that herbs can have on horses.

The research and practical experience gained in many years of hands on contact with the help and advice of some of the best trainers and veterinary surgeons in Europe, has ensured that Wendy and Terry Jennings are unique in their knowledge and experience in the benefits of feeding herbs to horses.

Wendy and Terry Jennings are the founders of Wendals Herbs. A family owned company that specialises in natural health care products for horses and dogs.

The information in this book has been gathered over many years of research and practical experience by the authors. They have personally fed herbs to hundreds of horses and prepared blends for many thousands of others.

This book is not intended for the diagnosis or treatment of horses which should always be supervised by a veterinary surgeon and no medicinal claim or advice is implied in this book.

INTRODUCTION

There are many books written on the subject of herbs. Most of them focus on the culinary or medicinal benefits to humans, or on how to grow them.

The purpose of this book is to give the reader an "easy to follow" guide to some of the herbs that are most commonly fed to horses, and the reasons why people have done so for many years.

In the United Kingdom we are required by law to ensure that an unwell horse receives the attention of a qualified veterinary surgeon and in all circumstances the authors would advise this. However, many ailments and behavioural problems in horses are avoidable with good feeding and management and herbs can often play their part in helping to maintain good all round well being in a horse. Many veterinary surgeons are now receptive to the medicinal benefits that some herbs have and are increasingly encouraging the use of them in the treatment of various conditions, sometimes after having tried a number of synthetic substances first.

Prevention is always better than cure and it is well known that nutrition is a major factor in maintaining good health. Feeding herbs can assist greatly.

DEDICATION

To our many equine friends, past and present, that have given us so much joy and sadness. We thank you for the pleasure you have given and for the opportunity of learning from you to benefit others.

THANKS

Our sincere thanks go to all those who have been so much help during the preparation of this book. In particular special mention must be given to "Legsley" for her many hours of typing, Dennis Hemmings for his artwork contribution and Nicola Jennings D.C. A.M.C. M.M.C.A. for her section on McTimoney Chiropractic treatment.

CONTENTS

	The Authors	3
	Introduction	5
Section One		
	A Brief Background to Herbs	11
	Choosing Herbal Products	13
	Feeding Herbs to Horses	15
	Feeding Guide	17
	Common Names	19
	Latin Names	21
Section Two		
	Materia Medica	23
Section Three		
	Herb Actions	109
	Vitamins and Minerals	119
	Other Herbal Preparations	127
	Aromatherapy	129
	Homeopathy	131
	Bach Flower Remedies	132
	McTimoney Chiropractic	133
Section four		
	The Digestive System	137
	The Respiratory System	153
	The Circulatory System	161
	The Urinary System	167
	The Coat and Skin	169
	The Muscular and Skeletal System	181
	The Reproductive System	193
	Behaviour	203
	Box Rest	211
	Eyes	212
Section Five		
	Useful Addresses	215
	Glossary	217
	Index	219

SECTION ONE

A Brief Background to Herbs	11
Choosing Herbal Products	13
Feeding Herbs to Horses	15
Feeding Guide	17
Common Names	19
Latin Names	21

A BRIEF BACKGROUND TO HERBS

The term herb refers to a plant, or plant part, that is used for its medicinal, savoury or aromatic qualities. There are hundreds of thousands of identified plants and probably even more that are yet to be discovered and named.

A plant may consist of leaves, roots, fruit, flowers, bark, stems or seeds and any part of these may contain the active ingredient that gives a plant its medicinal qualities.

Herbs have been used since very early times and it has long been recognised that they not only give nutritional benefits but they can also offer exceptional medicinal qualities. In years gone by they formed the basis for treating many ailments in both humans and animals. There were no synthetic drugs or patent medicines to turn to so great use was made of the natural growing plants.

As time passed herbs became very closely associated with medical practice and mans knowledge of some of the effects of them widened. During the 16th and 17th century two great herbalists, Gerrard and Culpeper, wrote much on the medicinal powers of herbs. Gardens were specifically planted with herbs for the expanding medical demands and many plants from other countries were found to be of great value.

As more herbs came to be used it was necessary for there to be a means of identifying the various types and to record international names, therefore in the mid 18th century all herbs were classified and given Latin names for reference, to assist the practising herbalist.

Whilst various herbal formulations were in constant use a new scientific approach began and chemical substitutes for valuable herbal extracts were developed. The manufacture of these artificial substances enabled scientists to make products that could be used for the treatment of ailments, without being dependent on the growing of the natural plants. This process formed the beginning of the mass production of medicines as we know them. Even today, the medical industry still uses an enormous amount of natural plants to produce medicines and drugs.

Horses are used and treated far differently to many years ago. We now set them many new tasks and have changed the way they live. They are no longer allowed to run in wild herds, or graze freely, to eat the various natural herbs and plants that grow. We control our horses far more and they have to be well mannered, well groomed and ready for the task that we set them.

Today most grazing is void of many of the herbs and plants that a horse would choose to eat naturally if he could. In an effort to maximise the production of lush grass we treat our paddocks to prevent the "weeds" from growing. It is interesting to note that when new paddocks are being laid at top stud farms a special mix is used which includes a number of herbal plants.

The horseman of yesteryear made great use of herbs. To a great extent our use decreased over the years because of the simplicity of buying medicines over the counter in neat packets and bottles. However the benefits of herbs have not gone away, and the gathering of top quality herbs is now made easier by the tremendous improvement in equipment and transport. It is now common to reduce the bulk and weight of herbs to a much more manageable product.

Herbs have recently been re-discovered. Wherever you look there is new recognition of their benefits. Several animal feed manufacturers are now adding herbs to their processed feeds and there are veterinary surgeons who specialise in using the treatment of herbal and other natural methods, rather than synthetic drugs.

Herbs are not a wonder cure and they will not cure every ailment or problem that exists, nor will drugs or other manufactured products. What herbs can do is assist in allowing the natural bodily functions to operate more efficiently. It is well known that herbs such as Chamomile help to relax the nervous system, whilst Garlic can help with alleviating respiratory disorders and repelling insects. These are simple examples of some of the recognised benefits that have been found with herbs over the many years since they were first "discovered".

CHOOSING HERBAL PRODUCTS

If you choose to feed herbs to your horse you have to decide if you are able to feed these fresh, dried or by using a product containing herbal extracts.

In an ideal world the herbs would be fresh but in most cases this is not practical, hence the enormous flood of "herbal" products to hit the market in recent years.

Extracts can be good, but having gone through that process they are usually diluted in varying amounts, according to the price and quality of the finished product.

Our preference is to feed good quality dried herbs. There is a wide range of these available from just about every part of the world. This gives the opportunity of obtaining each individual herb from the area that produces the best quality.

If you are feeding herbs, or a herbal blend, for a particular purpose, it is important that you have the right formula. There is much confusion in the market these days as more and more companies present their products using the in vogue "herbal" image. Whilst in many cases these are not harmful, they do not always offer the "natural" approach to well being that they may seem to. For example some horse feed companies produce what they call "herbal" feeds that smell appealing and may have pictures of herbs shown on their packaging or publicity. The reality is that in most cases the percentage of herbs added to the feedstuff is so low that they would have a negligible beneficial effect. The vitamins, minerals and trace elements in such feedstuff are the same artificial ones that such companies use in their other feeds.

Some companies have products that combine herbs or herb extracts with other artificial vitamins and minerals. Again this can be a marketing tool that is "jumping on the bandwagon" of the "natural" approach since many of the additives are synthetic. The best advice when buying a "herbal" product is to check exactly what you are getting on the label.

When buying a proprietary blend of herbs it is wise to stick to those that are established and known to work. If you are not happy with the results you should speak to the company concerned – it may be that you need something different and a good company will try to help.

There are some very good products available and it is reassuring to note that there is increasingly more control over this type of product. An organisation that has pioneered the way to ensure that good standards are achieved is the British Association of Holistic Nutrition and Medicine (BAHNM). This is an independent body who examine and monitor suitable products and where they reach an acceptable standard they are granted a BAHNM licence. The veterinary adviser to this Association is Christopher Day M.R.C.V.S., a leader in the field of alternative treatments.

FEEDING HERBS TO HORSES

Because horses are herbivores it is natural for them to eat herbs. In their natural environment horses graze and they would readily eat various herbs whilst they grow. Herbs such as **Comfrey**, **Red Clover** and even wild **Garlic** will often be sought out and eaten when they are available. However, even in the "good old days" not all useful herbs were growing in the green pastures since each require differing climates to be at their best. This has meant that traditionally herbs have been supplemented to the diet.

In most cases eating the required herbs whilst they grow is not an option, and we either have to grow them specifically or to obtain them from a specialist grower.

Herbs are now in such great demand that there is a world market geared at producing them in sufficient quantity and quality for both human and animal consumption. It is hardly practical to supply these in their fresh state in any quantity and in most cases they are dehydrated to reduce bulk and to preserve them further. If carried out correctly this process can reduce the weight of the herb greatly because up to 90% of the fresh weight can be moisture. It can be possible to retain most of the vitamin, mineral and medicinal qualities of 10 grams of fresh herbs in as little as 1 or 2 grams of dried herbs.

Clearly the advantages of using dried herbs are great and generally speaking it is this form that most people now feed to horses.

Dried Herbs – feeding guidelines

Feeding herbs is not an exact science and there are a number of factors that can affect the quantity that you might feed to a horse.

a. Firstly the quality of herbs can vary like any other agricultural product. The climate and care taken during growing, harvesting and preparation are big factors in determining the quality of the herbs, in the same way as they can be with the process of preparing hay. There are good and bad crops and the vitamin and mineral contents vary accordingly.
b. The physiological effect that herbs can have will vary in different

animals, in the same way that other medicines and drugs can have varying effects in different horses. Where a horse or pony may normally have say 20 gms of a particular herb, it is not uncommon for a similar one to require twice as much of that herb to show the same benefit. Conversely, a herb can have such a dramatic effect in some cases, that only a half measure is sufficient to achieve the desired results.

c. In order to establish a suitable amount to feed, it is important to take account of the size and weight of the individual horse. (see feeding guide, page 17).

Over the years that we have been feeding blends of dried herbs we have found that a daily feeding rate of up to 10 grams (0.35oz) per 100 kgs (220 lbs) bodyweight is normally about the correct amount. Normally a maximum of 50 grams (1.76ozs) is sufficient for a horse of 500 kgs (1100 lbs). Where individual herbs are fed the amount required is usually less (see individual herbs).

It can take some time for the actions of herbs to start to become apparent and where we have wanted to see improvement in a short time we have fed up to twice the "normal" amount for an initial period of a week or so until some benefit is noticeable, then reduced the amount according to bodyweight and the other factors.

Even at normal rates it is not unusual to see some improvement after feeding for as little as a week, although in other cases it can take 3 weeks or so before the benefits become noticeable. However, even if it is not apparent, the herbs may still be making some progress.

As a general rule you should look at the situation further if no change is detectable after feeding herbs for a month.

FEEDING GUIDE

This feeding guide is for where a number of herbs are blended and fed together. These amounts represent a total daily ration of all herbs. It is intended as an indication only, based on approximate size and bodyweights below.

For individual herbs refer to the recommendations under the respective herb where the dosage for each dried herb is given based on an average size horse of 500kg (1100 lbs) – Pages 25- 105

Height h.h.	Bodyweight kgs	lbs	Suggested total daily amount of dried herbs at 10 gms per 100 kg of bodyweight gms	ozs
12	230-290	507-639	20-30	0.7-1.06
13	290-350	639-771	30-35	1.06-1.23
14	350-420	771-926	35-40	1.23-1.41
15	420-520	926-1146	40-50	1.41-1.76
16	500-600	1102-1323	50	1.76
17	600-725	1323-1598	60	2.1

COMMON NAMES

Common Name	Latin Name
Alfalfa (Lucerne)	Medicago sativa
Aloe	Aloe barbadensis
Aniseed	Pimpinella anisum
Arnica	Arnica montana
Balm (Lemon Balm)	Melissa officinalis
Basil	Ocimum basilicum
Bladderwrack (Seaweed)	Fucus vesiculosis
Buckwheat	Polygonum fagopyrum
Burdock	Arctium lappa
Celery	Apium graveolens
Chamomile (German)	Matricaria chamomilla
Chaste Tree	Agnus castus
Cleavers (Clivers)	Galium aparine
Coltsfoot	Tussilago farfara
Comfrey	Symphytum officinale
Couch Grass	Agropyron repens
Damiana	Turnera aphrodisiaca
Dandelion	Taraxacum officinale
Devils Claw	Harpagophytum procumbens
Echinacea	Echinacea angustifolia
Eyebright	Euphrasia officinalis
Fennel	Foeniculum vulgare
Fenugreek	Trigonella foenum-graecum
Garlic	Allium sativum
Ginkgo	Ginkgo biloba
Golden Rod	Solidago virgaurea
Hawthorn	Crataegus oxyacantha
Hops	Humulus lupulus
Horehound (White)	Marrubium vulgare
Horsetail	Equisetum arvense
Lavender	Lavandula officinalis
Lime Tree	Tilia europaea
Liquorice	Glycyrrhiza glabra

Common Name	Latin Name
Marigold	Calendula officinalis
Marjoram	Origanum vulgare
Marshmallow	Althaea officinalis
Meadowsweet	Filipendula ulmaria
Milk Thistle	Silybum marianum
Mint (Peppermint)	Mentha piperita
Nettle	Urtica dioica
Parsley	Petroselinum crispum
Periwinkle	Vinca major
Psyllium	Plantago psyllium
Raspberry	Rubus idaeus
Red Clover	Trifolium pratense
Red Poppy	Papaver rhoeas
Rosehips	Rosa canina
Rosemary	Rosmarinus officinalis
Sage	Salvia officinalis
Saw Palmetto	Serenoa serrulata
Slippery Elm	Ulmus fulva
St Johns Wort	Hypericum perforatum
Strawberry	Fragaria vesca
Tea Tree	Melaleuca leucadendron
Thyme	Thymus vulgaris
Valerian	Valeriana officinalis
Vervain	Verbena officinalis
Willow (White)	Salix alba
Witch Hazel	Hamamelis virginiana
Wormwood	Artemisia absinthium
Yarrow	Achillea millefolium

LATIN NAMES

Latin Name	Common Name
Achillea millefolium	Yarrow
Agnus castus	Chaste Tree
Agropyron repens	Couch Grass
Allium sativum	Garlic
Aloe barbadensis	Aloe
Althaea officinalis	Marshmallow
Apium graveolens	Celery
Arctium lappa	Burdock
Arnica montana	Arnica
Artemisia absinthium	Wormwood
Calendula officinalis	Marigold
Crataegus oxyacantha	Hawthorn
Echinacea angustifolia	Echinacea
Equisetum arvense	Horsetail
Euphrasia officinalis	Eyebright
Filipendula ulmaria	Meadowsweet
Foeniculum vulgare	Fennel
Fragaria vesca	Strawberry
Fucus vesiculosis	Bladderwrack (Seaweed)
Galium aparine	Cleavers (Clivers)
Ginkgo biloba	Ginkgo
Glycyrrhiza glabra	Liquorice
Hamamelis virginiana	Witch Hazel
Harpagophytum procumbens	Devils Claw
Humulus lupulus	Hops
Hypericum perforatum	St Johns Wort
Lavandula officinalis	Lavender
Marrubium vulgare	Horehound (White)
Matricaria chamomilla	Chamomile (German)
Medicago sativa	Alfalfa (Lucerne)
Melaleuca leucadendron	Tea Tree
Melissa officinalis	Balm (Lemon Balm)
Mentha piperita	Mint (Peppermint)

Latin Name	Common Name
Ocimum basilicum	Basil
Origanum vulgare	Marjoram
Papaver rhoeas	Red Poppy
Petroselinum crispum	Parsley
Pimpinella anisum	Aniseed
Plantago psyllium	Psyllium
Polygonum fagopyrum	Buckwheat
Rosa canina	Rosehips
Rosmarinus officinalis	Rosemary
Rubus idaeus	Raspberry
Salix alba	Willow (White)
Salvia officinalis	Sage
Serenoa serrulata	Saw Palmetto
Silybum marianum	Milk Thistle
Solidago virgaurea	Golden Rod
Symphytum officinale	Comfrey
Taraxacum officinale	Dandelion
Thymus vulgaris	Thyme
Tilia europaea	Lime Tree
Trifolium pratense	Red Clover
Trigonella foenum-graecum	Fenugreek
Turnera aphrodisiaca	Damiana
Tussilago farfara	Coltsfoot
Ulmus fulva	Slippery Elm
Urtica dioica	Nettle
Valeriana officinalis	Valerian
Verbena officinalis	Vervain
Vinca major	Periwinkle

SECTION TWO

Materia Medica

ALFALFA
Also known as **Lucerne**

Latin Name: Medicago sativa

Part Used: Leaves

Collection:
A perennial plant that grows 12" to 18" high, flowers in summer months.

Actions:
Alterative, Anthelmintic, Appetizer, Diuretic, Galactogogue, Nervine, Tonic, Vermifuge.

Usage:
A nutritious plant extensively fed to horses for its general tonic and nutritional qualities. It can also be helpful in cases of water retention and urinary infections

Authors comments:
Alfalfa is often used as a high fibre fodder. It is rich in calcium, potassium, magnesium, iron and many other vitamins and minerals.

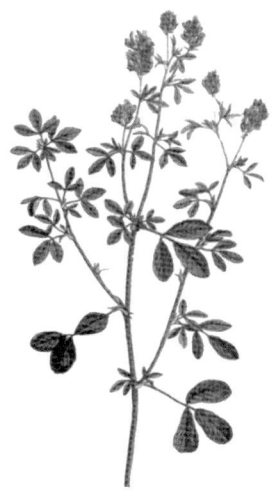

ALOE

Latin Name: Aloe barbadensis

Part used: Fresh leaves, stems and dehydrated juice from the leaves

Collection:
Aloes are indigenous to East and South Africa. They have also been introduced and extensively cultivated in the West Indies.

Actions:
Anthelmintic, Emmenagogue, Hepatic, Laxative, Vermifuge, Vulnerary.

Usage:
Internally - Used as a powerful laxative for constipation. In small doses it supports the oestrus cycle.

Externally - For minor burns, bites, skin irritations, sores and bruises.

Combinations:
When used internally to regulate the oestrus cycle it should be combined with calmatives to reduce griping.

Authors comments:
A member of the Lily family with fleshy leaves. There are over 200 species of Aloe, of which Aloe Vera is the most commonly used.

Aloe Vera has been marketed aggressively world wide and is used in a whole range of products from cosmetics to medicinal. Some commercially produced gels are unreliable because they can vary in purity and contain solvents which can cause an allergic reaction.

Warning:
Aloe Vera can stimulate the uterus and should be avoided during pregnancy.

ANISEED

Latin Name: Pimpinella anisum

Part Used: Seeds

Collection:
Originally from Egypt. Aniseed grows to 18" high and is collected from July to September.

Actions:
Antiseptic, Antispasmodic, Aromatic, Carminative, Diuretic, Expectorant, Galactogogue, Pectoral, Stimulant, Stomachic, Tonic.

Usage:
Internally – Used for digestive disorders, flatulence, colic, coughing and respiratory problems and for increasing milk flow.

Externally - The volatile oil is used for lice and other parasites.

Combinations:
Can be mixed with Fennel to help prevent colic.
Coltsfoot and Horehound combine well for severe coughing.

Dosage: 20 – 30 gms. Added to daily feed.

Authors comments:
This herb can be helpful in stimulating appetite and assisting in digestive disorders that could lead to colic symptoms. It is commonly used in respiratory blends. Avoid infusions during pregnancy.

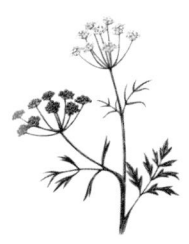

ARNICA

Latin Name: Arnica montana

Part Used: Flower

Collection:
Grown throughout Central Europe and gathered between June- August.

Actions:
Anti-inflammatory, Stimulant, Vulnerary.

Usage:
Helps relieve pain and reduce swelling from bruises, sprains and muscle strains.

Authors Comments:
Arnica is used in homeopathic preparations only for internal use and as a tincture or cream externally.

Warning:
The herb should not be taken internally.

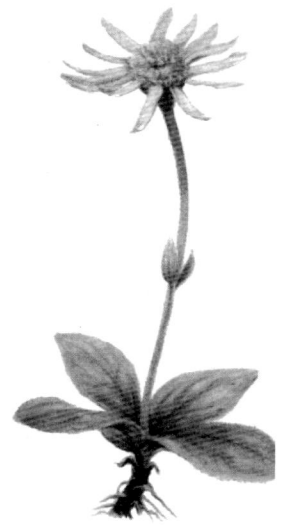

Arnica
Arnica montana

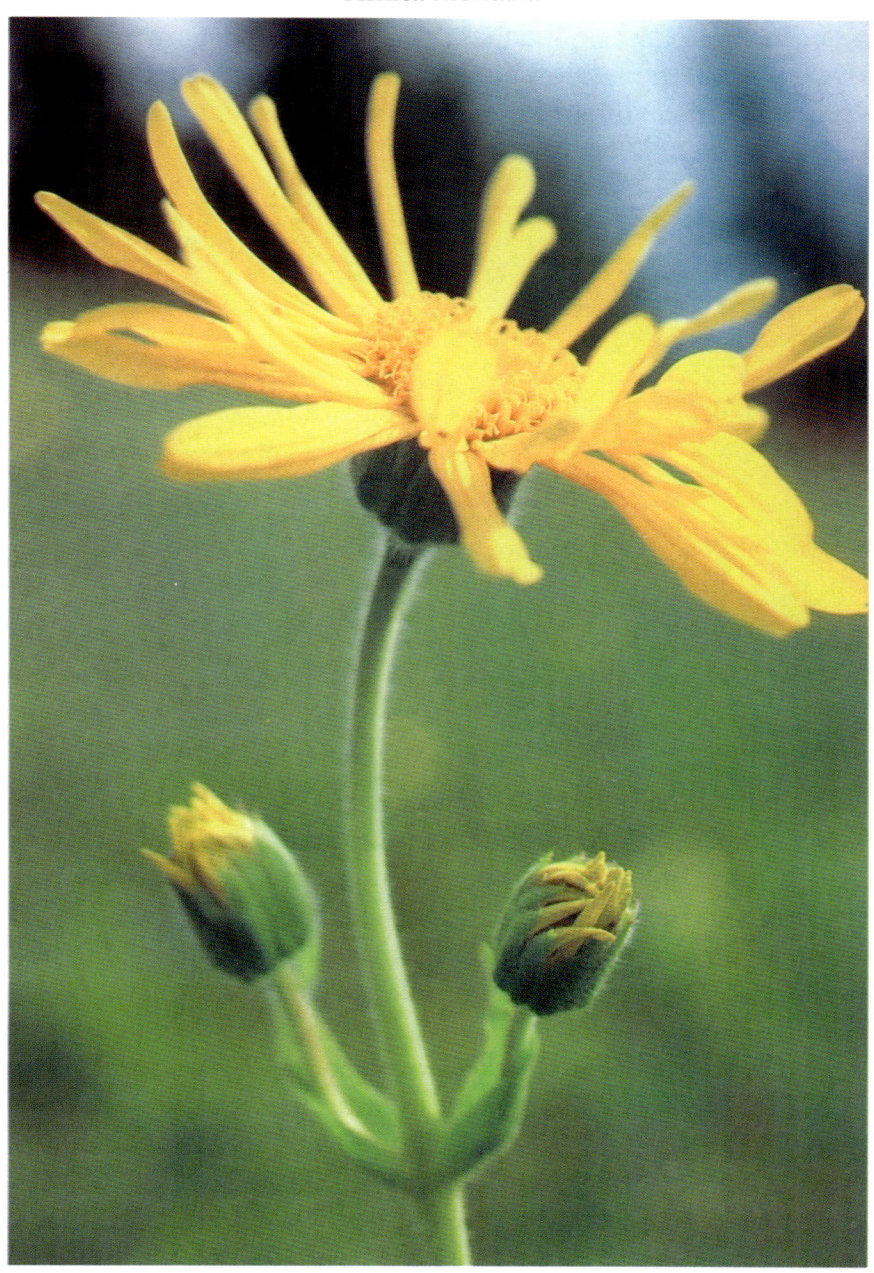

BALM
Also known as **Lemon Balm**

Latin Name: Melissa officinalis

Part Used: Leaves

Collection:
A native of the Mediterranean region that has now been widely introduced elsewhere. The leaves are collected before or after flowering between June and September.

Actions:
Antispasmodic, Aromatic, Bitter, Calmative, Carminative, Diaphoretic, Emmenagogue, Febrifuge, Nervine, Sedative, Stomachic, Tonic.

Usage:
A tonic that can be useful for female disorders, relieves cramps and helps regularise the oestrus cycle. It can help with digestive and nervous problems.

Combinations:
For digestive problems combine with Hops, Chamomile and Meadowsweet.

Dosage: 40 – 50 gms. Added to daily feed

Authors comments:
Can be helpful in regularising the oestrus cycle in mares and the associated discomfort.

Balm
Melissa officinalis

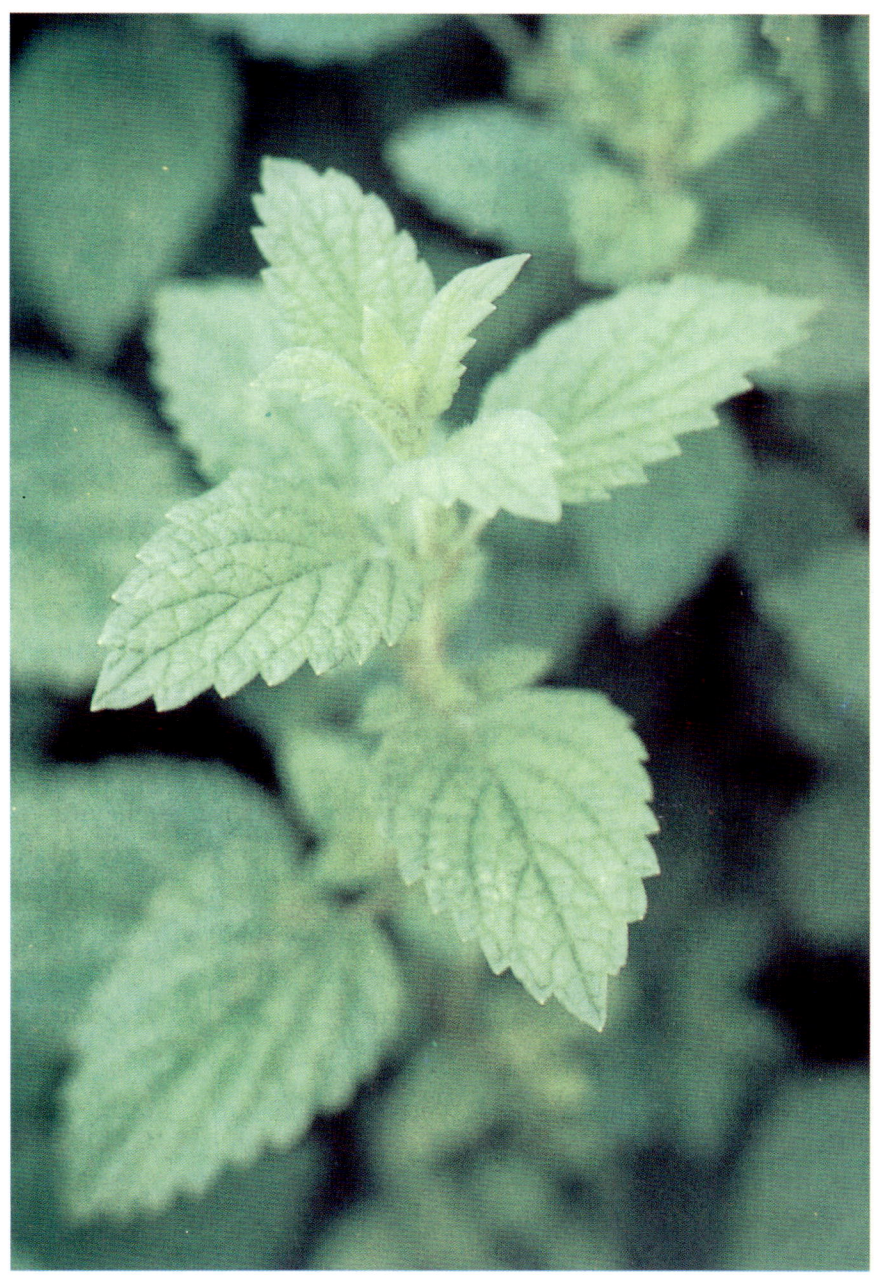

BASIL

Latin Name: Ocimum basilicum

Part Used: Herb

Collection:
A native of southern Asia and the Middle East although it is now grown commercially in Central and Southern Europe. Harvested throughout summer months.

Actions:
Antibacterial, Antifungal, Antispasmodic, Aromatic, Carminative, Expectorant, Galactogogue, Mild Sedative, Stomachic.

Usage:
Internally – Used for respiratory disorders such as coughs and for constipation or digestive disorders.

Externally - Can be used in a poultice and applied to itching skin and ringworm, using its bacteria and fungus fighting qualities.

Dosage: 40 – 50 gms. Added to daily feed.

Authors comments:
Basil is not used as commonly for medicinal purposes these days as it used to be, but it remains a useful herb for both internal and external use.

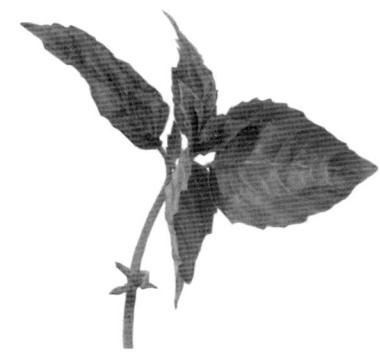

BLADDERWRACK
Also known as **Kelp** and **Seaweed**

Latin Name: Fucus vesiculosis

Part Used: Whole Plant

Collection:
Gathered from where the sea is pollution free. Available from a variety of countries including the west coast of Ireland.

Actions:
Alterative, Antibiotic, Antihypothyroid, Antirheumatic, Demulcent, Diuretic, Emmolient, Mucilage, Sedative, Stimulant, Tonic.

Usage:
Helps to stimulate an under-active thyroid gland. It is good for coat and hoof conditions and an aid to arthritic and rheumatic conditions.

Dosage: 40 – 50 gms. Added to daily feed.

Authors comments:
Bladderwrack, or dried seaweed, is an original source of iodine. It is also rich in calcium, magnesium, potassium, selenium and many other vitamins. Seaweed is sometimes used as a fertilizer due to its potash content which helps promote growth of grass whilst remaining safe for horses to graze. It is thought to reduce obesity through stimulating the thyroid gland.

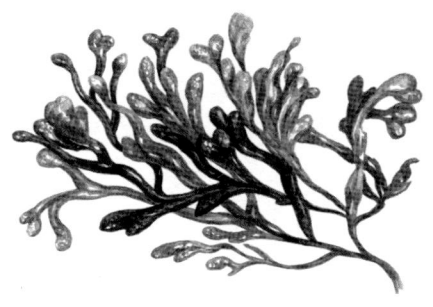

BURDOCK

Latin Name: Arctium lappa

Part Used: Root

Collection:
Grown throughout Europe. The roots of first year plants are collected before flowering in July.

Actions:
Alterative, Antimicrobial, Antiseptic, Aperient, Bitters, Cholagogue, Diaphoretic, Diuretic, Laxative, Mucilage, Tonic, Vulnerary.

Usage:
Internally - For skin complaints, arthritis, rheumatism, blood disorders, liver tonic.

Externally - Can be made into a wash for ulcers, boils and ringworm.

Dosage: 20 gms. Added to daily feed.

Authors comments:
A very effective "blood cleanser" probably best known for its benefits for skin problems. This herb is also helpful in taking away excess fluid and reducing swelling.

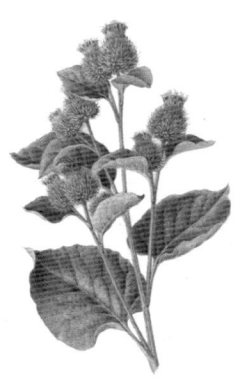

Burdock
Arctium lappa

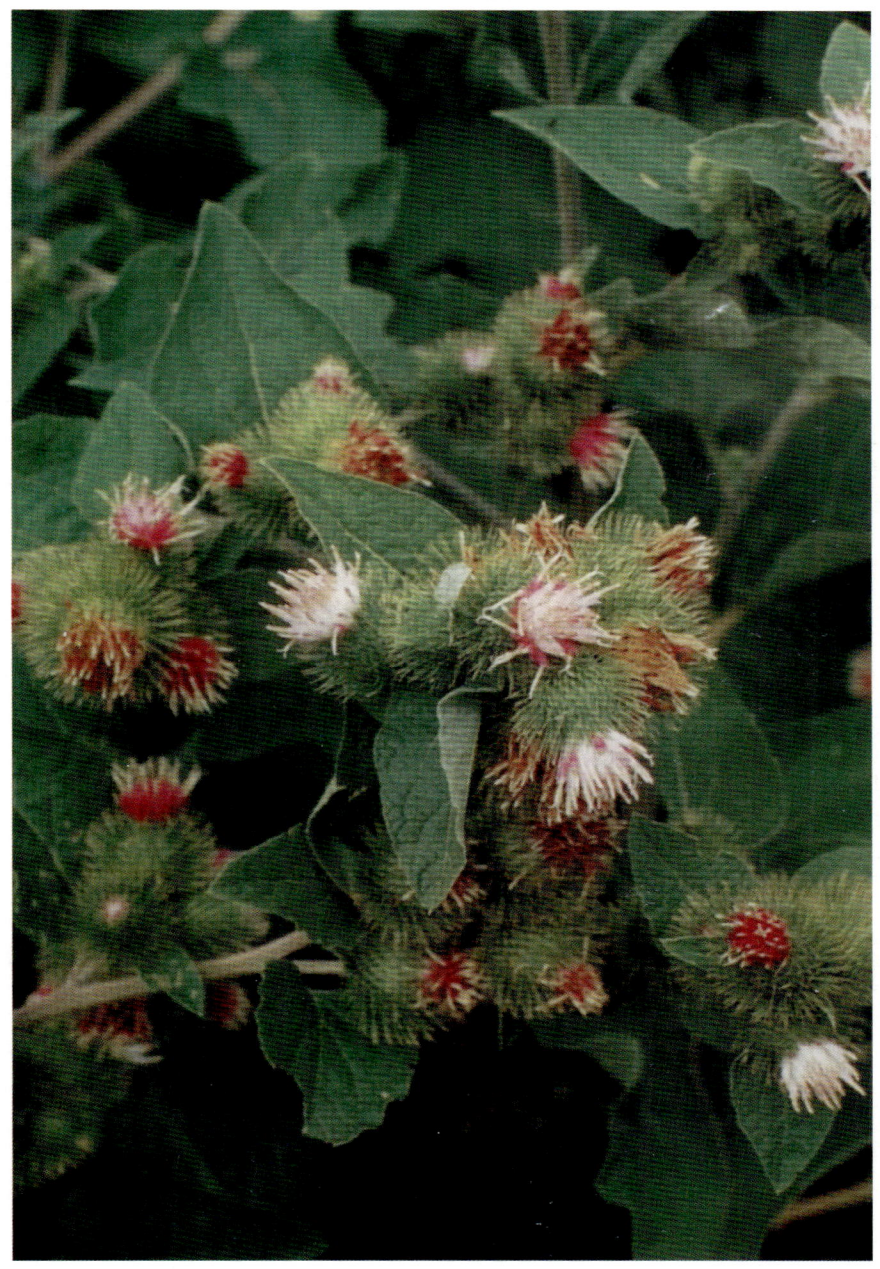

BUCKWHEAT

Latin Name: Polygonum fagopyrum

Part Used: The fruit

Collection:
A native of Northern or Central Asia. Cultivated in the United States. The fruit is collected whilst in flower.

Actions:
Acrid, Antihistamine, Astringent.

Usage:
Circulatory disorders. Can help strengthen and repair capillaries and is helpful in conditions relating to poor circulation.

Dosage: 40 – 50 gms. Added to daily feed.

Authors comments:
Contains rutin, a substance that effects the strength and permeability of the capillary walls.

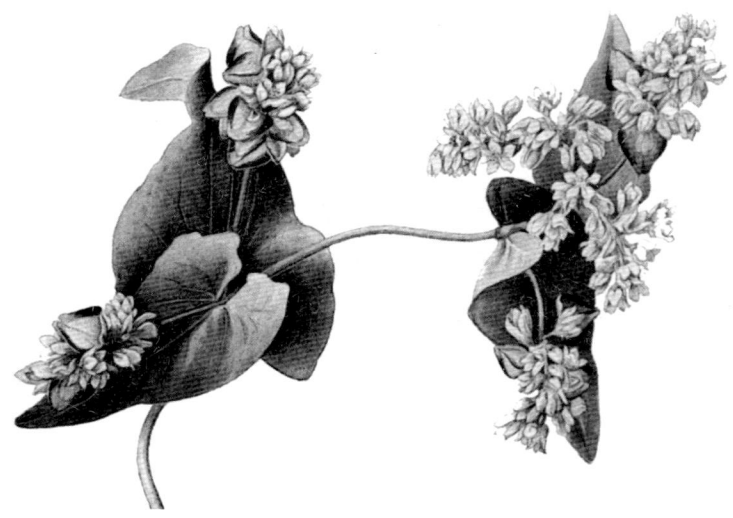

CELERY

Latin Name: Apium graveolens

Part used: Seeds, herb and root

Collection:
Grows in Europe, the United States of America and Africa. Collected from June to September.

Actions:
Alterative, Anti-inflammatory, Antiseptic, Aromatic, Bitters, Carminative, Diuretic, Hepatic, Nervine, Sedative, Stimulant, Stomachic, Tonic.

Usage:
The seed is particularly good for rheumatism and arthritis. It also assists the process of digestion.

Combinations:
Combines with Dandelion for rheumatic conditions.

Dosage: 15 – 20 gms. Added to daily feed.

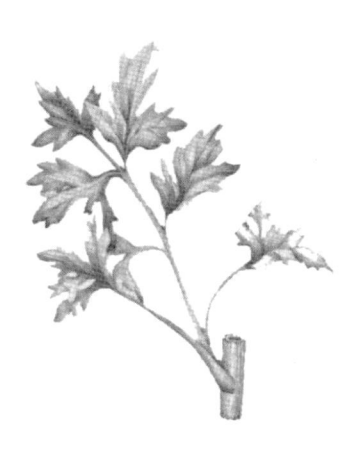

CHAMOMILE (GERMAN)

Latin Name: Matricaria chamomilla

Part used: Flowers

Collection:
Collect flowers from May to August and gently dry at moderated temperature.

Actions:
Alterative, Analgesic, Anodyne, Anti-inflammatory, Antiseptic, Antispasmodic, Aromatic, Bitter, Calmative, Carminative, Diaphoretic, Emmenagogue, Laxative, Mucilage, Nervine, Sedative, Stomachic, Tonic, Vulnerary.

Usage:
Internally – Feed for stress, tension and nervous conditions and those associated with digestive disorders. Also helpful for menstrual cramps.

Externally – Can be applied in liquid form to wounds, bruises and skin disorders.

Combinations:
With other sedative herbs to make a calming and relaxing blend.

Dosage: 30 – 40 gms. Added to daily feed.

Authors comments:
Chamomile is best known for its relaxing qualities and can be helpful for both horse and rider for nervous tensions before competing. It will not adversely affect the performance. A bunch of the flowers hanging in the stable is said to help deter the flies.

Chamomile
Matricaria chamomilla

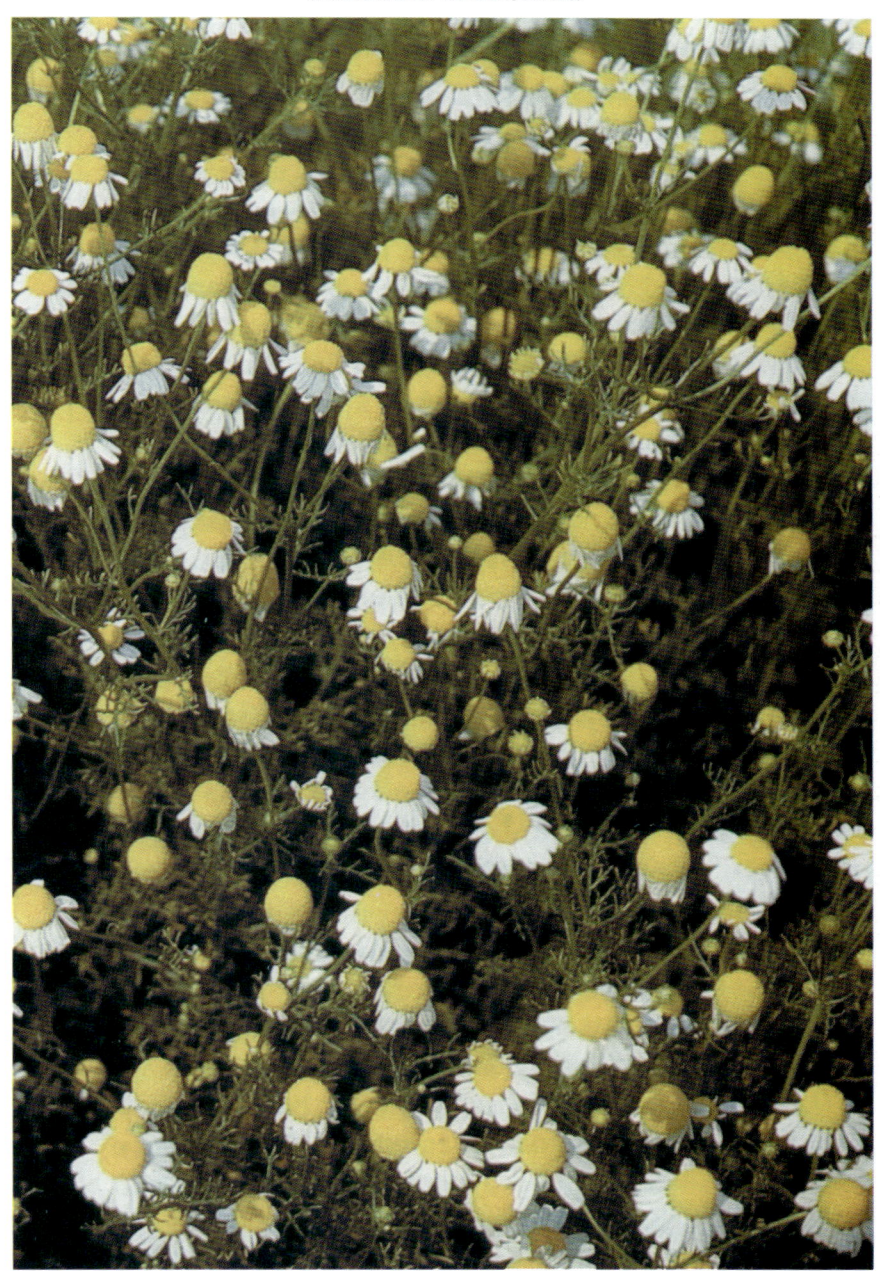

CHASTE TREE
Also known as **Monks Pepper**

Latin Name: Agnus castus

Part Used: Fruit

Collection:
Grown on the shores of the Mediterranean. The berries are picked when ripe in October and November.

Actions:
Aromatic, Carminative, Emmenagogue, Restorative, Sedative, Tonic.

Usage:
For PMT (PMS) and in cases of hormonal disorders.

Dosage: 30 gms. Added to daily feed.

Authors comments:
Chaste Tree Berries are regarded as a hormonal normaliser and they help to regulate the oestrus cycle. Therefore they can be a useful aid in preparing a mare for covering as well as relieving the effects of PMT (PMS). Chaste Tree Berries can also be helpful in male horses by helping to normalise irregular behaviour resulting from hormonal disorder.

Warnings:
Do not use during pregnancy.

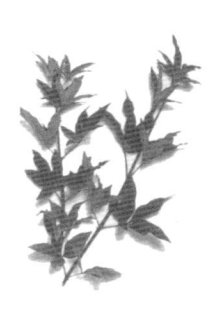

CLEAVERS (CLIVERS)
Also known as **Goose Grass**

Latin Name: Galium aparine

Part Used: Herb

Collection:
Abundant as a hedgerow weed throughout Europe and North America. Gathered in March to May when just coming into flower.

Actions:
Alterative, Antiseptic, Antispasmodic, Aperient, Astringent, Diuretic, Laxative, Tonic, Vulnerary.

Usage:
Internally - Skin diseases and irritations, urine infections, soft swellings and fluid retention.

Externally - Healing wounds.

Dosage: 40 – 50 gms. Added to daily feed.

Authors comments:
This herb has a reputation of having curative qualities for growths and tumours. An excellent tonic for the lymphatic system. Rich in calcium, copper, iodine and sodium.

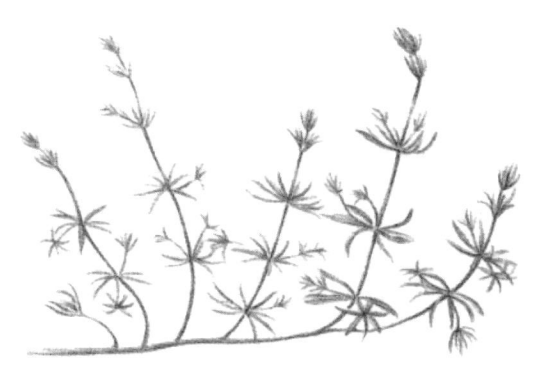

COLTSFOOT

Latin Name: Tussilago farfara

Part Used: Dried flowers and leaves

Collection:
A native of Europe, including the UK. Gather before fully bloomed and dry in shade. Collect flowers from February to April. Collect leaves from May to June.

Actions:
Anticatarrhal, Astringent, Bitter, Demulcent, Diuretic, Emollient, Expectorant, Mucilage, Pectoral, Tonic.

Usage:
Respiratory problems, including coughing, asthma and pneumonia. Also used for diarrhoea and as a general tonic.

Combinations:
Horehound and Marshmallow can be combined for ailments of the respiratory system.

Dosage: 20 – 30 gms. Added to daily feed.

Authors comments:
Historically this herb was one of the most popular cough remedies for humans. It is still used as the principal herb for herbal tobacco where it is said to relieve the respiratory system.

Warnings:
There is some controversy in the medical world as to whether large amounts of this herb can cause liver problems. It should be avoided in pregnant or nursing mares.

Coltsfoot
Tussilago farfara

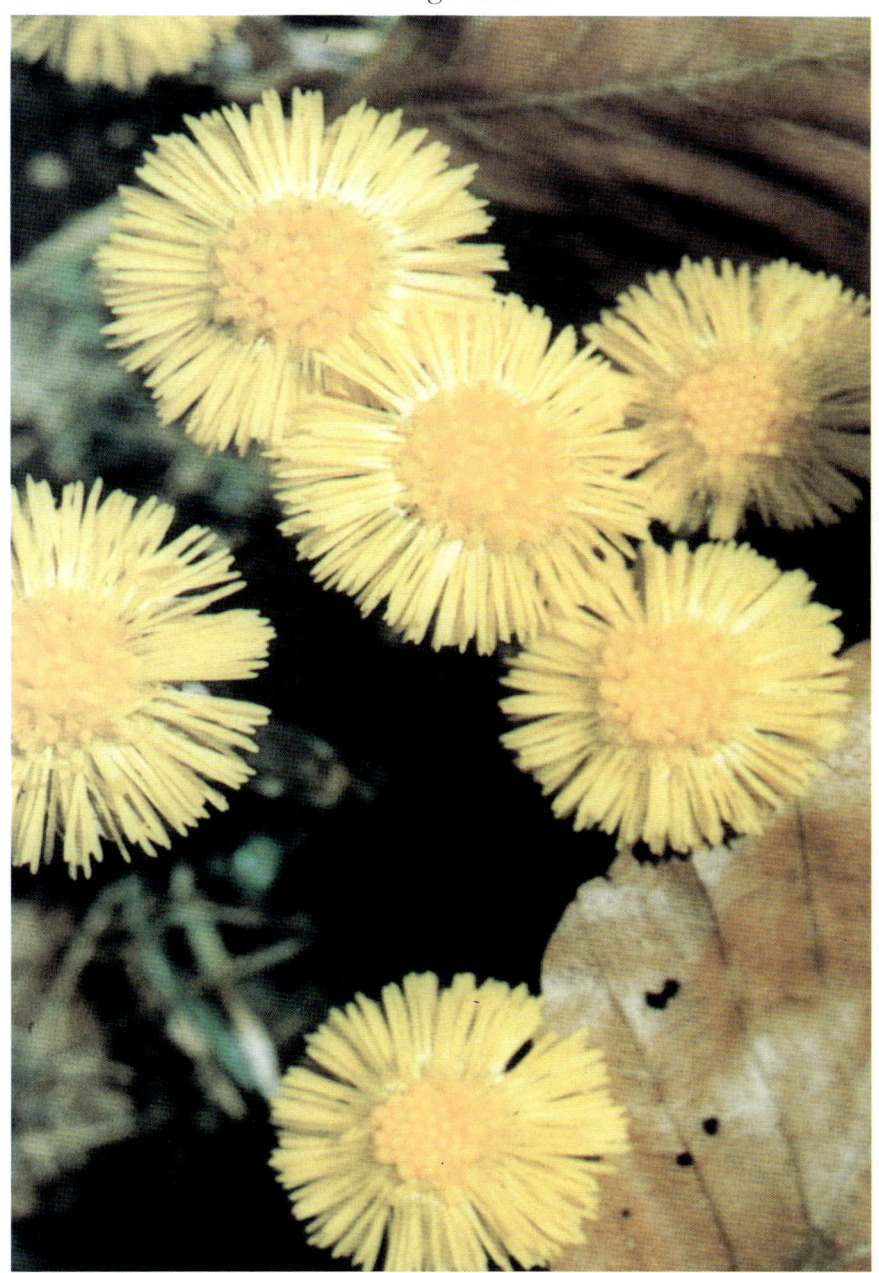

COMFREY
Also known as **Knitbone**

Latin Name: Symphytum officinale

Part Used: Leaves and roots

Collection:
A native of Europe it is widespread throughout the UK on riverbanks and ditches. Collect spring and summer. Flowers May to June.

Actions:
Anti-inflammatory, Astringent, Demulcent, Emollient, Expectorant, Haemostatic, Mucilage, Pectoral, Tonic, Vulnerary.

Usage:
Internally - To encourage healing of bone and tissue. Good for respiratory conditions, arthritis, rheumatism, diarrhoea and bleeding.

Externally - Wounds, sprains and as a poultice for boils and abscesses.

Combinations:
For respiratory problems Coltsfoot and Horehound. For ulcers and inflammation Marshmallow and Meadowsweet are suitable.

Dosage: 40 – 50 gms. Added to daily feed.

Authors comments:
Comfrey is an excellent herb to promote the healing of bone and tissue. For a fracture or severe injury that needs help to heal quickly there is no better herb. The healing qualities can help in repairing damage to lungs and the respiratory system when a horse "bleeds" or "bursts". Used correctly we believe Comfrey to be an excellent aid to healing.

Warnings:
There has been some controversy over possible liver damage that may result from feeding large quantities over a long period of time.

COUCH GRASS

Latin Name: Agropyron repens

Part Used: The Rizome or underground stem

Collection:
Grows in Northern Africa and Europe. Collected March and April also August and September and separated from leaves and roots. Dried and chopped.

Actions:
Antibiotic, Antilithic, Antimicrobial, Aperient, Demulcent, Diuretic, Laxative, Mucilage, Tonic, Vermifuge.

Usage:
Used for disorders of the urinary tract and kidney infections. A mild laxative.

Dosage: 40 – 50 gms. Added to daily feed.

Authors comments:
The tenacious growing Couch Grass is a common nuisance to farmers and gardeners alike. The medicinal qualities are not always appreciated. In humans it is reputed to be helpful for gout and rheumatism. Dogs and cats may eat the leaves to promote vomiting. It also acts as a mild laxative.

DANDELION
Known as **Wet the Bed**

Latin Name: Taraxacum officinale

Part Used: Root or leaves

Collection:
A native of Europe. Root is collected June to August, leaves are collected anytime.

Actions:
Alterative, Antirheumatic, Aperient, Bitter, Cholagogue, Diuretic, Hepatic, Laxative, Stimulant, Stomachic, Tonic.

Usage:
Internally – For water retention, inflammation, kidney and liver complaints including jaundice. Stimulates appetite and aids digestion. Also used for rheumatism, arthritis, laminitis and is a mild laxative.

Externally - The pressed juice from stalks or leaves can be an effective cure for warts.

Dosage: 40 – 50 gms. Added to daily feed.

Authors comments:
An extremely effective diuretic herb that has the benefit of replacing lost potassium. Dandelion is one of the most useful of native British medicinal herbs as all parts of the plant are effective and safe to use.

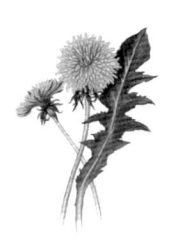

Dandelion
Taraxacum officinale

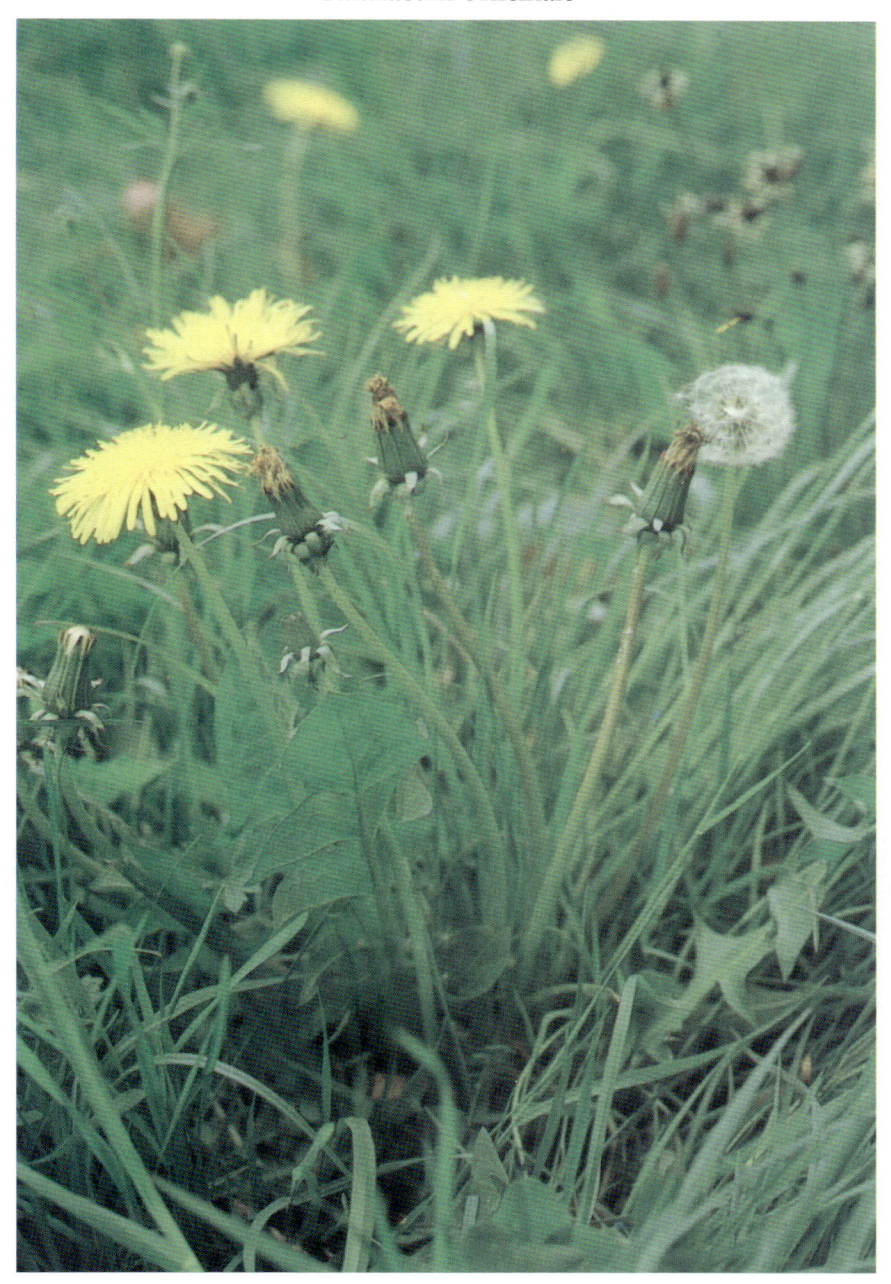

DAMIANA

Latin Name: Turnera aphrodisiaca

Part Used: Leaves and stem

Collection:
Gather when flowering. Habitat: Mexico, South America, Texas, West Indies.

Actions:
Antidepressant, Aphrodisiac, Bitter, Laxative, Nervine, Stimulant, Tonic.

Usage:
Strengthens nervous system. Increases sexual drive.

Dosage: 10 – 20 gms. Added to daily feed.

Authors comments:
Alkaloids which contain a testosterone like action (male hormone) which could be helpful in increasing sexual drive are contained in Damiana.

Warnings:
There are other herbs such as Aplopappul, Bigelovia, Veneta (known as Damiano False) which have different constituents.

DEVILS CLAW

Latin Name: Harpagophytum procumbens

Part Used: Root

Collection:
Indigenous to Southern and Eastern Africa. Roots are collected at the end of the rainy season.

Actions:
Analgesic, Anodyne, Anti-inflammatory, Antirheumatic, Bitter, Diuretic, Sedative.

Usage:
For arthritis, rheumatism, degenerative joint disorder (DJD) and to reduce inflammation and pain.

Dosage: 40 – 50 gms. Added to daily feed.

Authors comments:
Devils Claw is now looked upon as a natural alternative to Phenylbutazone (Bute) and Cortisone, since it has similar actions. There are no apparent adverse side effects. Many companies now produce Devils Claw in a liquid form often with other ingredients. As in all products, some are better than others.

Warnings:
Devils Claw is a uterine stimulant and should not be fed to pregnant mares.

ECHINACEA

Latin Name: Echinacea augustifolia

Part Used: Leaves and roots

Collection:
A native of America. Cultivated in Britain. Collected in September and October.

Actions:
Alterative, Antibacterial, Antibiotic, Anticatarrhal, Anti-inflammatory, Antimicrobal, Antiseptic, Antiviral, Aphrodisiac, Immuno-stimulant, Tonic.

Usage:
Increases bodily resistance against viral and bacterial infection.

Dosage: 40 – 50 gms. Added to daily feed.

Authors comments:
This is an excellent herb for the prevention and cure of viral and bacterial infections. It has the effect of enhancing the immune system by stimulating the production of white blood cells.

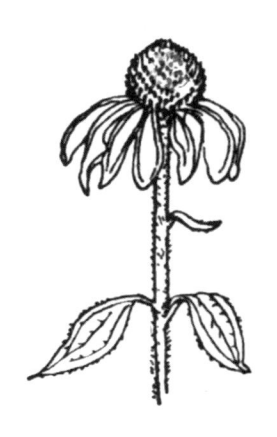

Echinacea
Echinacea augustifolia

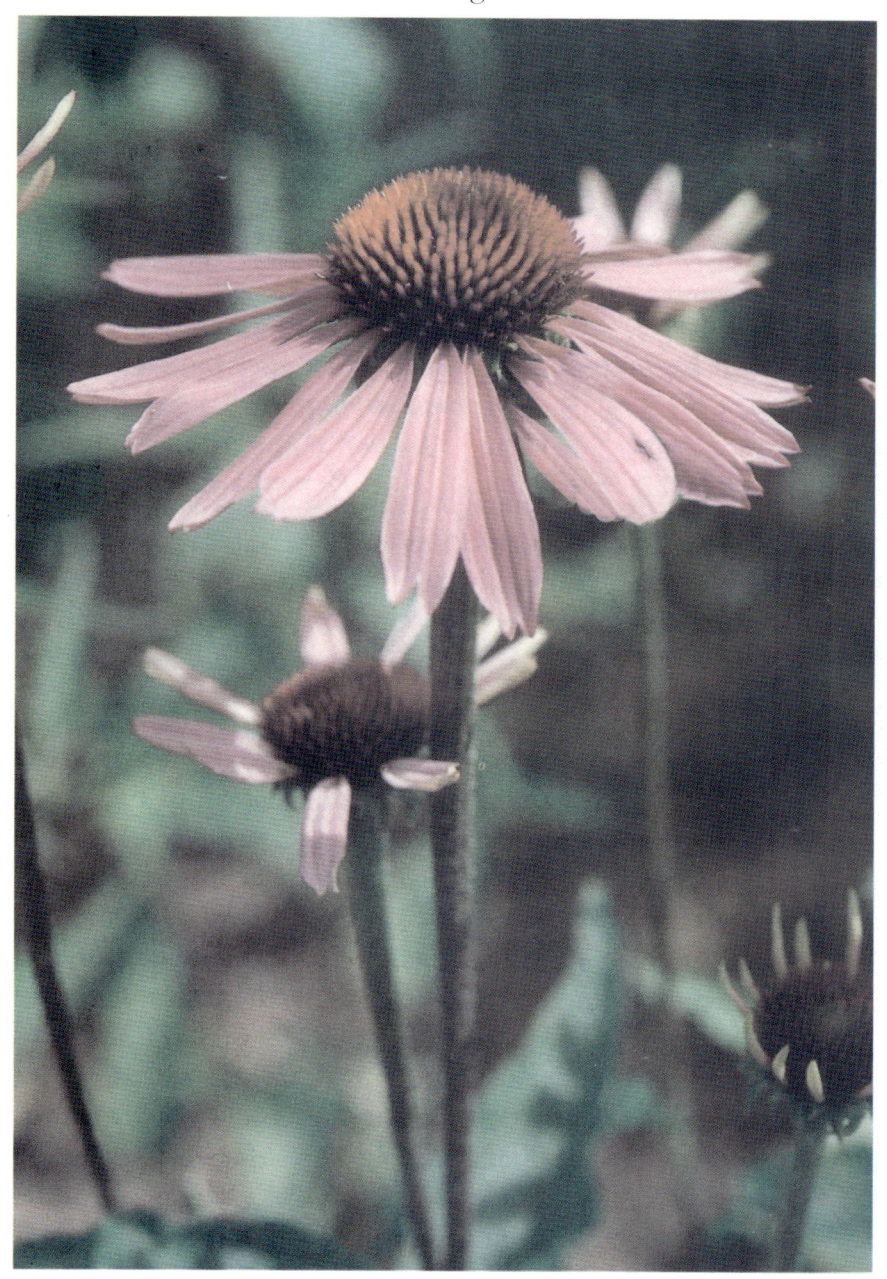

EYEBRIGHT

Latin Name:: Euphrasia officinalis

Part Used: Whole plant

Collection:
Relatively common in damp meadows and woods throughout the British Isles. Best collected in August and up to October when in full flower.

Actions:
Anticatarrhal, Anti-inflammatory, Antiseptic, Astringent, Bitter, Nervine, Stomachic, Tonic.

Usage:
Internally – Suitable for feeding to stimulate the liver. Also can be fed for nasal congestion and catarrh.

Externally – Can be used as a lotion for the eyes where it is useful for its qualities.

Dosage: 30 – 40 gms. Added to daily feed.

Authors comments:
Used in herbal tobacco for chronic bronchial colds.

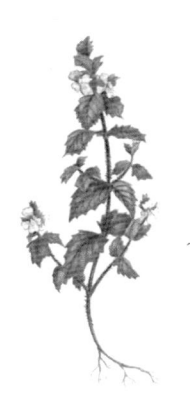

FENNEL

Latin Name: Foeniculum vulgare

Part Used: Seeds

Collection:
A native of the Mediterranean but will thrive anywhere. Collected between August and October.

Actions:
Antiseptic, Antispasmodic, Aromatic, Carminative, Diuretic, Expectorant, Galactogogue, Hepatic, Mucilage, Rubefacient, Stimulant, Stomachic, Tonic.

Usage:
Coughs, appetite, constipation, diarrhoea and stimulates milk flow in nursing mares. Also good for urinary disorders due to its qualities as a mild diuretic.

Combinations:
Mixes well with other herbs for respiratory problems such as Garlic, Liquorice and Red Clover. Fennel oil with honey makes a good cough remedy.

Dosage: 30 – 40 gms. Added to daily feed.

Authors comments:
A decoction can be used as an eyewash for irritations and strains. Fennel is disliked by fleas and in a powdered form helps keep them away from stables and kennels. Chewing the seed helps bad breath.

Warnings:
Avoid high doses during pregnancy.

FENUGREEK

Latin Name: Trigonella foenum-graecum

Part Used: Seed

Collection:
In Autumn. Indigenous to the Eastern Mediterranean. Cultivated in India, Africa, Egypt and Morocco.

Actions:
Aphrodisiac, Appetizer, Aromatic, Carminative, Demulcent, Disinfectant, Emollient, Expectorant, Galactagogue, Laxative, Mucilage, Restorative, Stomachic, Tonic, Vulnerary.

Usage:
Internally - As a conditioner it stimulates digestion. Useful for coughs and as a general tonic. It also helps to stimulate milk flow.

Externally - The crushed seeds can be used for bruises, swellings, boils and ulcers.

Combinations:
Often combined with Garlic for general use.

Dosage: 40 – 50 gms. Added to daily feed.

Authors comments:
Very good for stimulating appetite and improving condition. Increases milk flow in the nursing mare.

To make a paste for external use, crushed seeds can be mixed in hot milk – allow to cool before use.

Warnings:
Avoid large quantities in early pregnancy. Also in mares with hormonal problems, where it can sometimes affect their behaviour.

GARLIC

Latin Name: Allium sativum

Part Used: Bulb

Collection:
Originally from India or Asia. Garlic is now cultivated throughout the world. It is collected July - September.

Actions:
Alterative, Anthelmintic, Antibiotic, Anticatarrhal, Antihistamine, Antimicrobal, Antiseptic, Antispasmodic, Antiviral, Aromatic, Carminative, Cholagogue, Diaphoretic, Diuretic, Expectorant, Febrifuge, Mucilage, Pectoral, Rubefacient, Stimulant, Tonic, Vermifuge, Vulnerary.

Usage:
Internally - Commonly used to repel flies and insects. Helps with coughs and respiratory disorders, rheumatism, aids digestion and intestinal infections.

Externally - Can be applied for bites, ringworm or boils.

Dosage: 40 – 50 gms. Added to daily feed.

Authors comments:
The best known herb most commonly used for horses which has many qualities and benefits. It helps prevent coughs, improves digestion and prevents worms. Also Garlic promotes sweating and in doing so excretes through the skin to repel flies and insects. Although Garlic can taint the milk in a lactating mare it transfers its benefits to the foal.

Many "Garlic powders" on the market are not pure Garlic and the quality is questionable. Pure Garlic Granules are best to work with.

GOLDEN ROD

Latin Name: Solidago virgaurea

Part Used: Aerial parts

Collection:
Harvest between July and October. Found throughout Britain, Europe and the United States.

Actions:
Anticatarrhal, Antifungal, Anti-inflammatory, Antiseptic, Antispasmodic, Aromatic, Astringent, Carminative, Diaphoretic, Diuretic, Expectorant, Stimulant, Vulnerary,

Usage:
Internally - Kidney and bladder disorders, flatulence and digestive problems and for coughs and asthma.

Externally - As a poultice or ointment for ulcers and slow healing wounds.

Combinations:
Can be mixed with Echinacea and used for respiratory problems.

Dosage: 40 – 50 gms. Added to daily feed.

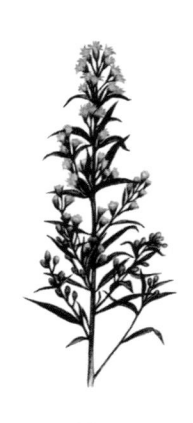

Golden Rod
Solidago virgaurea

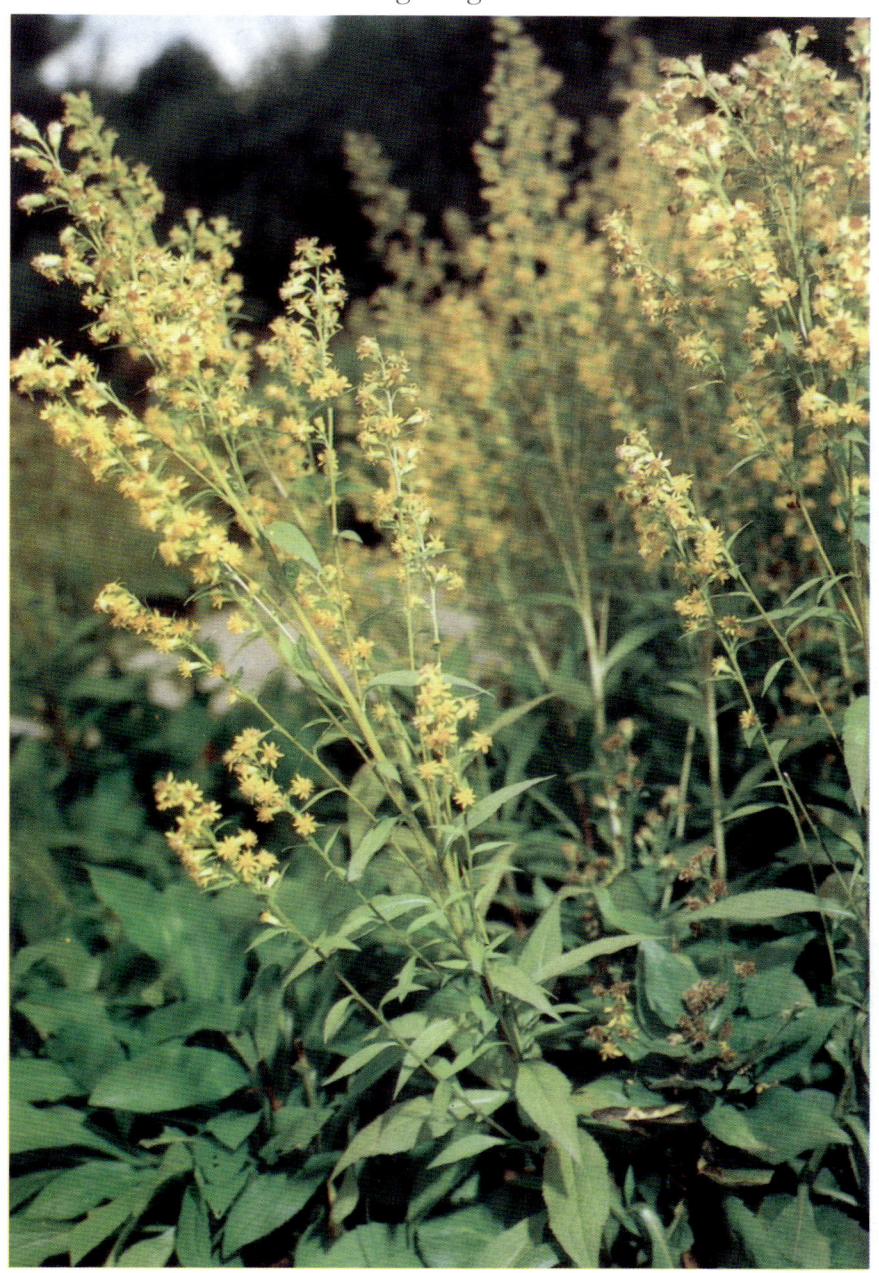

GINKGO

Latin Name: Ginkgo biloba

Part Used: Leaves and seeds

Collection:
A native of China which has been produced in Europe since the early 1700's. The leaves are collected during autumn months.

Actions:
Antifungal, Astringent, Bitter, Expectorant, Nervine, Sedative.

Usage:
Improves circulation and blood flow throughout the body. Good for coughs and allergies. Believed to be helpful for growths.

Dosage: 30 – 40 gms. Added to daily feed.

Authors Comments:
Ginkgo is an antioxidant which means it slows the formation of free radicals which are believed to be responsible for cancer.

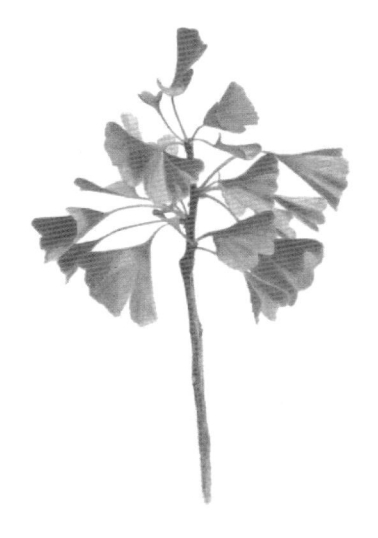

HOPS

Latin Name: Humulus lupulus

Part Used: Flowers

Collection:
Before fully ripened during August or September. Grown in some parts of England, mainly Kent as well as the U.S.A., Germany, France, South Russia and Australia.

Actions:
Analgesic, Antiseptic, Antispasmodic, Anodyne, Astringent, Bitter, Diuretic, Febrifuge, Hypnotic, Nervine, Sedative, Stimulant, Stomachic, Tonic, Vermifuge.

Usage:
Calming, nervous diarrhoea, stimulates appetite, digestive ailments.

Combinations:
Combines well with Valerian Root for excitable, nervous and spasmodic conditions.

Dosage: 20 – 30 gms. Added to daily feed.

Authors Comments:
The bitter taste of Hops makes some horses pick at them, but as part of a calming blend they are very effective, particularly in colts.

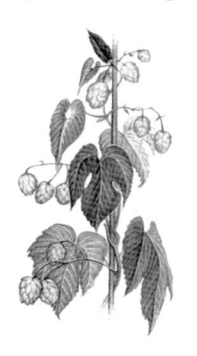

HAWTHORN

Latin Name: Crataegus oxyacantha

Part Used: Dried haws or berries

Collection
September and October. Common in Britain, Europe and the U.S.A.

Actions:
Antispasmodic, Astringent, Cardiac, Diuretic, Sedative, Tonic.

Usage:
A general tonic for the heart, lowers high blood pressure and aids digestion.

Dosage: 15 – 20 gms. Added to daily feed.

Warning: Do not feed to pregnant mares.

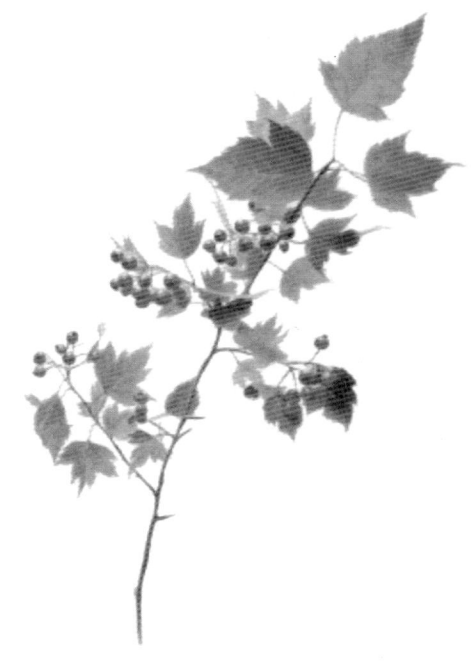

Hawthorn
Crataegus oxyacantha

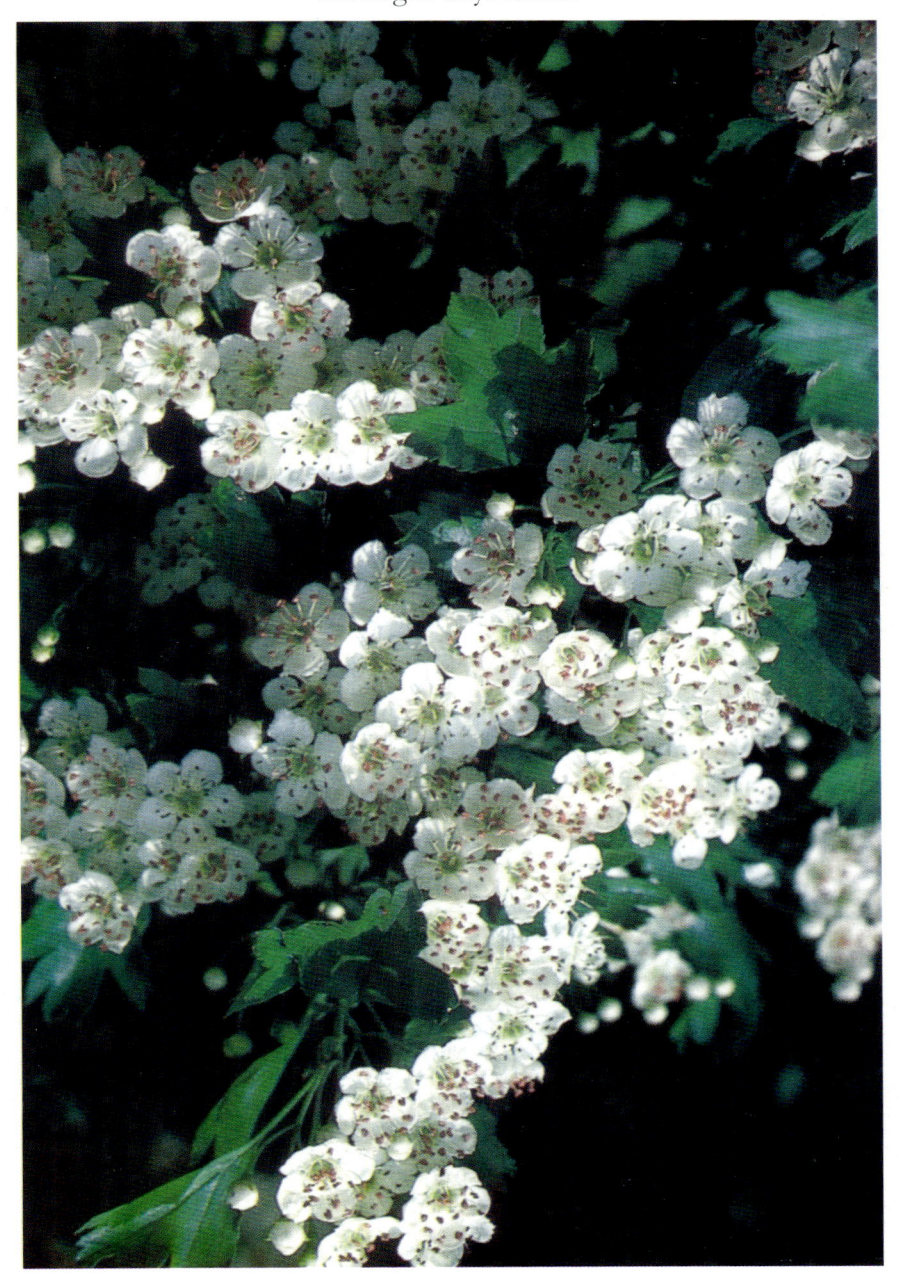

HOREHOUND (WHITE)

Latin Name: Marrubium vulgare

Part Used: The herb

Collection:
Grows throughout various parts of Europe including East Anglia in the UK. Harvested between June to September.

Actions:
Antispasmodic, Aromatic, Bitter, Cholagogue, Diaphoretic, Diuretic, Emmenagogue, Expectorant, Pectoral, Sedative, Stimulant, Stomachic, Tonic, Vulnerary,

Usage:
For coughs and respiratory conditions. An effective digestive stimulant and a tonic that is particularly good for inflammation of the liver and jaundice.

Combinations:
Combines well with Liquorice and Marshmallow for severe respiratory conditions.

Dosage: 30 – 40 gms. Added to daily feed.

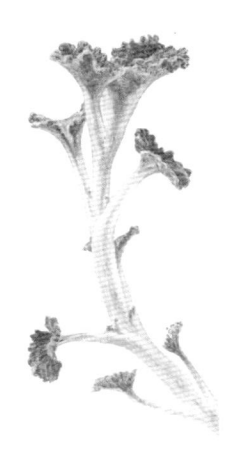

HORSETAIL

Latin Name: Equisetum arvense

Part Used: Stems

Collection:
Native to the British Isles where it is widespread in fields and wasteground of light sandy soil. The green stems are the medicinal parts. Collected from May to July.

Actions:
Astringent, Carminative, Diuretic, Emmenagogue, Galactagogue, Haemostatic, Vulnerary.

Usage:
Internally - Used for kidney and bladder disorders and to help arrest internal and external bleeding. Also beneficial for arthritis.

Externally - For bleeding wounds and healing.

Warnings:
Like many herbs Horsetail has toxic characteristics and whilst it can be beneficial in small doses, caution should be taken. Used correctly this powerful herb can form part of an effective herbal blend. It is best avoided in pregnant mares.

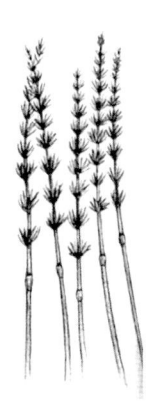

LAVENDER

Latin Name: Lavandula officinalis

Part Used: Flowers

Collection:
A vigorous growing plant that grows in various countries from Europe to as far away as Australia. Before flowers open in summer months.

Actions:
Antidepressant, Antimicrobal, Antiseptic, Antispasmodic, Carminative, Cholagogue, Diuretic, Nervine, Relaxant, Rubefacient, Sedative, Stimulant, Stomachic, Tonic.

Usage:
For nervous ailments and as a relaxant.

Dosage: 20 – 30 gms. Added to daily feed.

Authors comments:
The oil is used extensively in perfumes and toiletries.

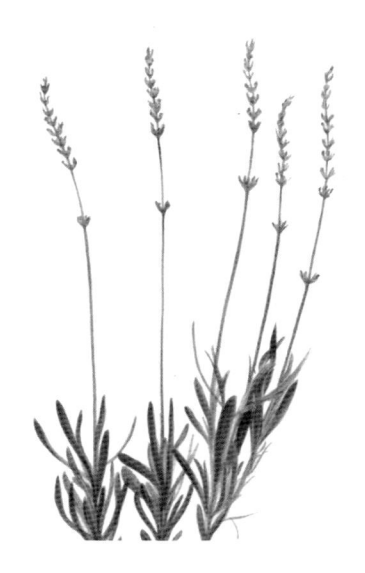

Lavender
Lavandula officinalis

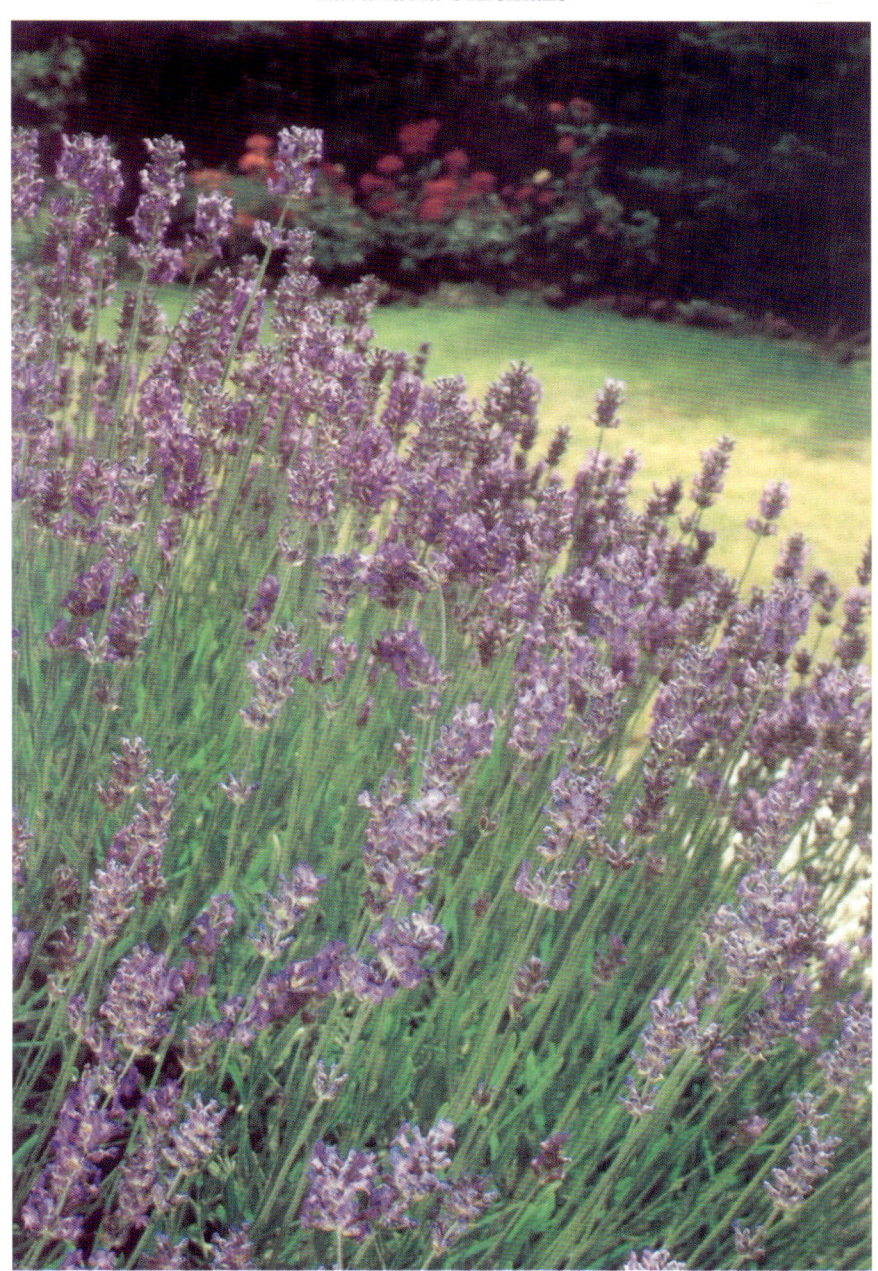

LIME TREE

Latin Name: Tilia europaea

Part Used: Flowers

Collection:
Grows throughout the West Indies and a native of Asia. Collected immediately after they have flowered in mid summer.

Actions:
Alterative, Anti-inflammatory, Antispasmodic, Astringent, Diaphoretic, Diuretic, Expectorant, Mucilage, Nervine, Tonic.

Usage:
Used for nervous ailments, colds, fevers and as an aid to PMT (PMS) type behaviour in mares.

Combinations:
For nervous tension combine with Hops.

Dosage: 20 – 30 gms. Added to daily feed.

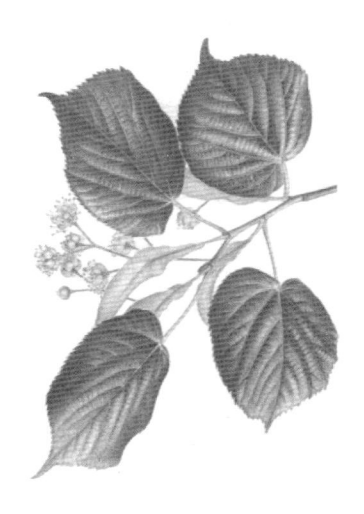

LIQUORICE

Latin Name: Glycyrrhiza glabra

Part used: Root

Collection:
Extensively grown in South East Europe and South West Asia. The roots are not ready to take up and use until the third season. Harvesting normally occurs in the autumn of the fourth year.

Actions:
Alterative, Antibacterial, Anti-inflammatory, Antispasmodic, Antiviral, Aphrodisiac, Demulcent, Diuretic, Emollient, Expectorant, Laxative, Pectoral, Relaxant, Stomachic, Tonic.

Usage:
For arthritis, bladder ailments, coughs and as a general tonic. It is also a digestive aid in the prevention of colic.

Combinations:
As a mild laxative combined with Fennel. With Coltsfoot or Horehound for coughs.

Dosage: 20 – 30 gms. Added to daily feed.

Warnings:
Not recommended for pregnant and nursing mares.

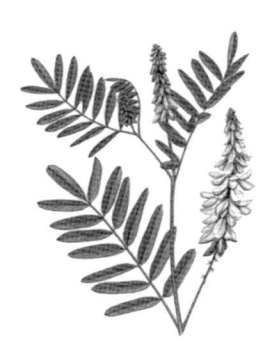

MARIGOLD

Latin Name: Calendula officinalis

Part used: Flowers and petals

Collection:
A native of Southern Europe but grows well in the UK. Flowers can be collected throughout summer months.

Actions:
Alterative, Analgesic, Antibacterial, Antidepressant, Anti-inflammatory, Antifungal, Antimicrobial, Antiseptic, Antispasmodic, Aperient, Aromatic, Astringent, Bitter, Cholagogue, Diaphoretic, Diuretic, Emmenagogue, Febrifuge, Mucilage, Stimulant, Tonic, Vermifuge, Vulnerary.

Usage:
Internally - Particularly beneficial for skin problems and as an aid to digestion. It also helps induce perspiration and to regulate the oestrus cycle.

Externally - Used as a lotion or cream for sprains, wounds and swellings.

Combinations:
With Marshmallow for digestion, with Cleavers and Nettles for skin complaints.

Dosage: 30 – 40 gms. Added to daily feed.

Warning:
Do not feed during pregnancy.

Marigold
Calendula officinalis

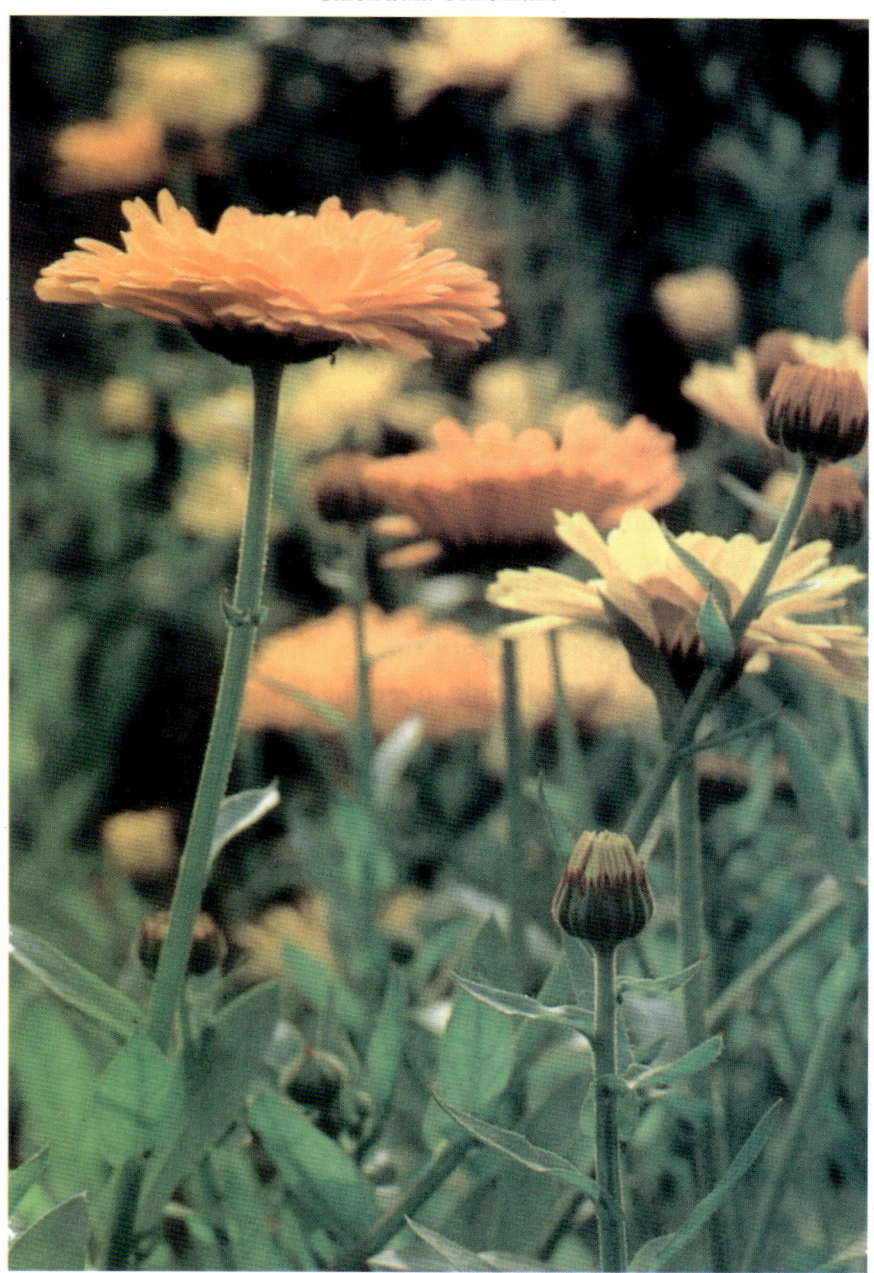

MARJORAM

Latin Name: Origanum vulgare

Part Used: Herb

Collection:
A native to Europe. It is collected as soon as it flowers from the wild in the Mediterranean region, as well as being cultivated commercially in many countries.

Actions:
Alterative, Antiseptic, Antispasmodic, Aromatic, Astringent, Bitter, Calmative, Carminative, Diaphoretic, Emmenagogue, Expectorant, Nervine, Rubefacient, Stimulent, Stomachic, Tonic.

Usage:
For digestive disorders including diarrhoea. Also used for coughs.

Dosage: 30 – 40 gms. Added to daily feed.

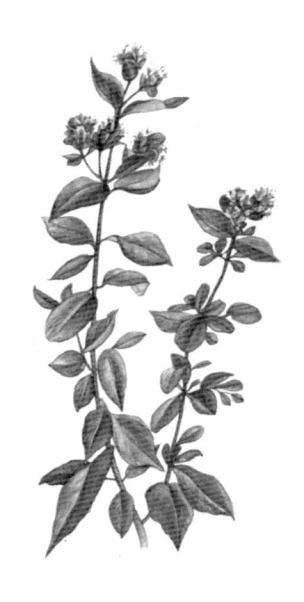

MARSHMALLOW

Latin Name: Althaea officinalis

Part Used: Root and leaves

Collection:
Native to the British Isles and widespread from Western Europe to Siberia. Collect leaves in summer after flowering. Roots in autumn.

Actions:
Astringent, Demulcent, Diuretic, Emollient, Expectorant, Galactagogue, Laxative, Mucilage, Pectoral, Tonic, Vulnerary.

Usage:
Internally - Used for urinary complaints, stomach and intestinal disorders and coughs.

Externally - As a poultice.

Dosage: 30 – 40 gms. Added to daily feed.

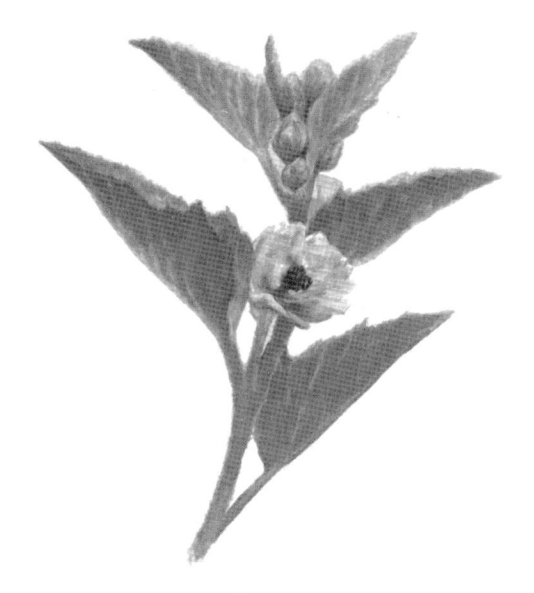

MEADOWSWEET

Latin Name: Filipendula ulmaria

Part Used: Herb

Collection:
Common in damp woods and meadows throughout Europe. Collected throughout summer months when the flowers are fully opened.

Actions:
Alterative, Antacid, Anti-inflammatory, Antipyretic, Antirheumatic, Antiseptic, Antispasmodic, Aromatic, Astringent, Diuretic, Mucilage, Stomachic, Tonic.

Usage:
For rheumatic and arthritic pain, bladder and kidney disorders and reducing fever.

Dosage: 40 – 50 gms. Added to daily feed.

Authors comments:
Contains salicylic acid, the substance from which acetylsalicylic acid (aspirin) was synthesised.

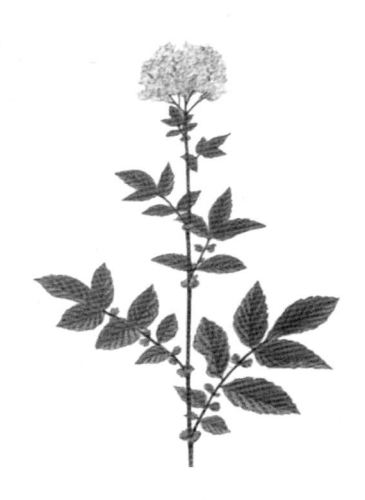

Meadowsweet
Filipendula ulmaria

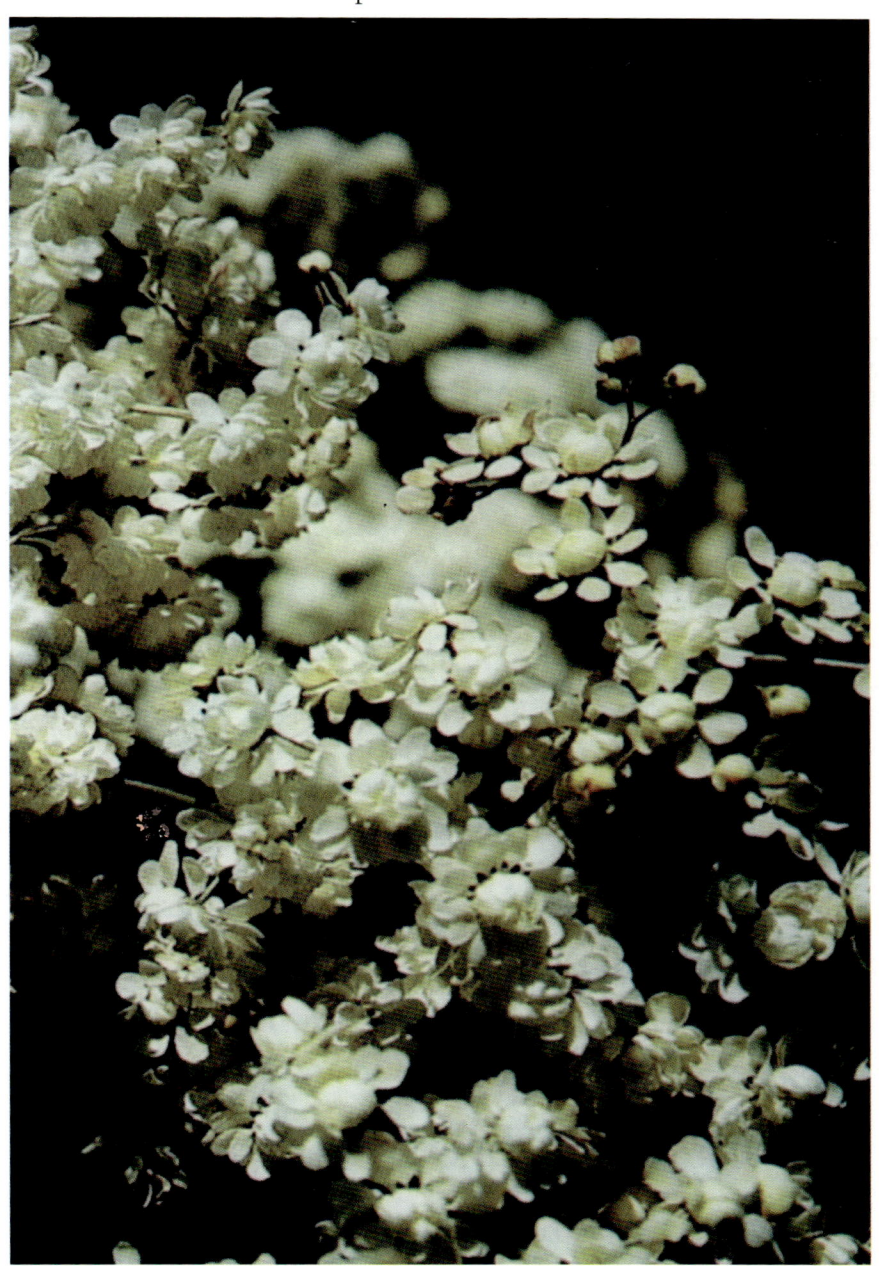

MILK THISTLE

Latin Name: Silybum marianum

Part Used: Seeds

Collection:
A native of Southern Europe but it has been widely introduced elsewhere. Flowers in summer months when the seed heads are cut and stored for a couple of days then shaken to remove seeds.

Actions:
Bitter, Cholagogant, Demulcent, Galactogogue, Nervine, Stimulant, Tonic.

Usage:
Best known as a liver tonic it detoxifies poisons that enter the blood stream. It also promotes milk production

Dosage: 20 – 30 gms. Added to daily feed.

Authors Comments:
Used in the pharmaceutical industry for processing into tinctures and tablets which are used medicinally for gall bladder disease and the regeneration of tissue in cases of liver damage.

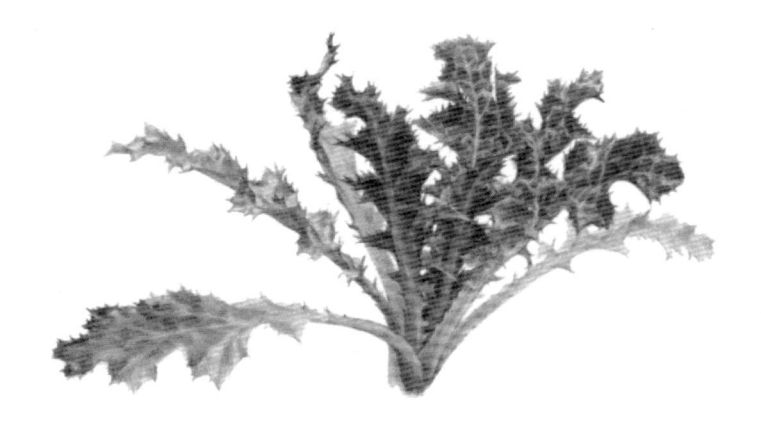

MINT
Also known as **Peppermint**

Latin name: Mentha piperita

Part Used: Leaves

Collection:
Cut just before flowering from the end of July to the end of August in England. A second crop can be obtained in September.

Actions:
Alterative, Analgesic, Antibacterial, Anticatarrhal, Anti-inflammatory, Antimicrobial, Antiseptic, Antispasmodic, Antiviral, Anodyne, Aromatic, Astringent, Calmative, Carminative, Diaphoretic, Febrifuge, Nervine, Rubefacient, Sedative, Stimulent, Stomachic, Tonic.

Usage:
An aid to the digestive system in the prevention of flatulence, diarrhoea and colic. It also induces perspiration and can help coughs,

Dosage: 30 – 40 gms. Added to daily feed.

Authors comments:
Used as an appetiser to help encourage the horse to eat and its strong pleasant smell makes it ideal to add to feed. It can be helpful in drying up a lactating mare.

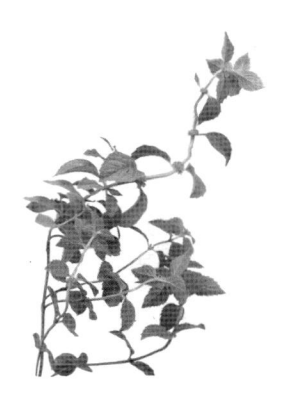

NETTLES

Latin Name: Urtica dioica

Part Used: Aerial parts

Collection:
Grows extensively throughout Europe and the U.K. Best used when in bloom.

Actions:
Alterative, Antiseptic, Astringent, Diuretic, Expectorant, Galactagogue, Haemostatic, Rubefacient, Stimulent, Tonic.

Usage:
Haemorrhaging, anaemia, rheumatism, arthritis, laminitis, sweet itch, spring tonic, allergies, milk production, appetite, coat and skin.

Dosage: 40 – 50 gms. Added to daily feed.

Authors comments:
Provides iron and vitamin C to help strengthen and enhance the circulatory system. Helps in the elimination of waste products through the functions of the liver and kidneys. An extremely good blood tonic that can "quicken the spirit" particularly in a thoroughbred.

Warnings:
Occasionally a horse can develop a nettle rash in which case it might be better avoided.

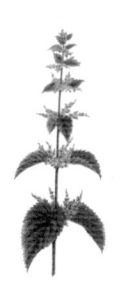

Nettles
Urtica dioica

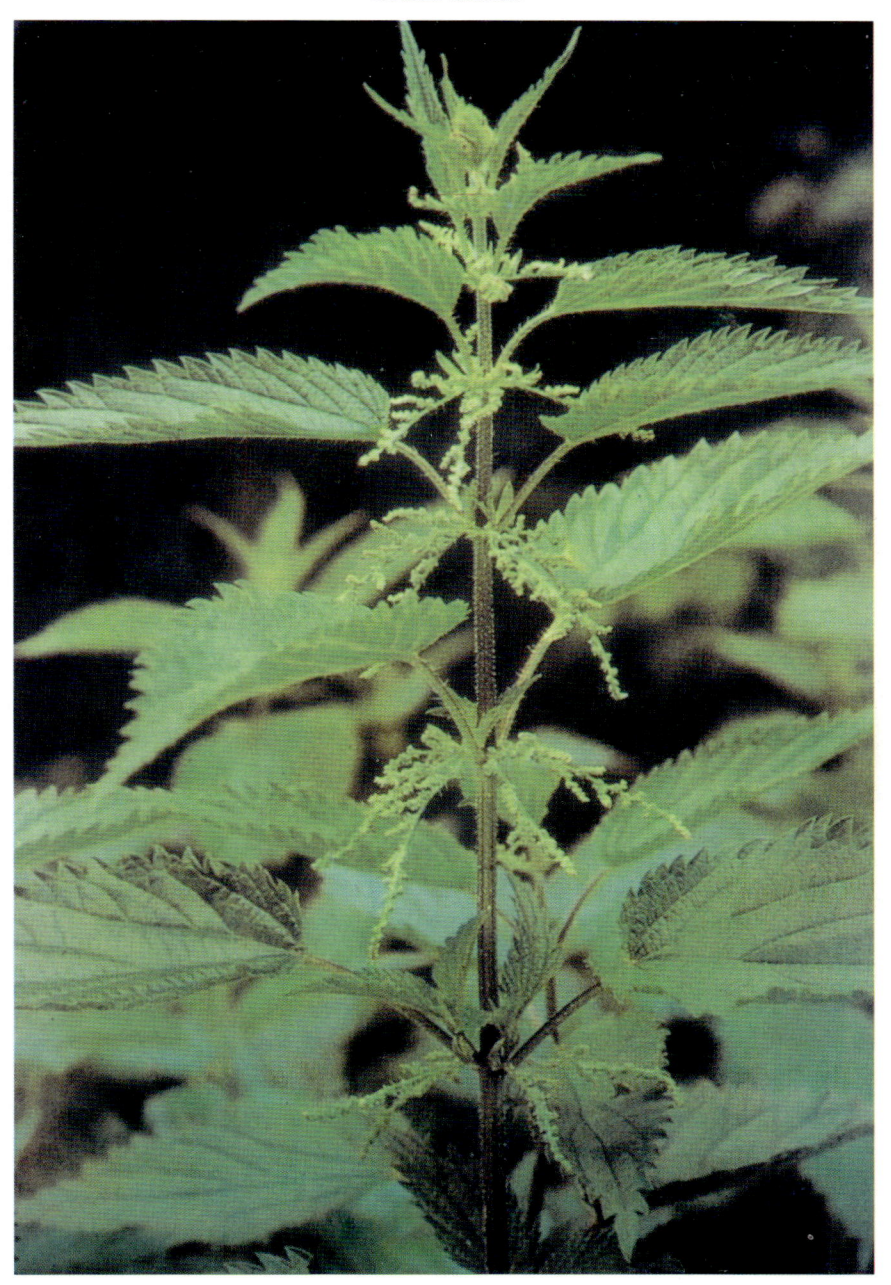

PARSLEY

Latin Name: Petroselinum crispum

Part Used: Leaves, root and seeds

Collection:
Traditionally grown in Eastern Mediterranean countries and brought to England in the 16th century. Leaves when growing, roots from second year plants.

Actions:
Antihistamine, Antirheumatic, Antiseptic, Antispasmodic, Aperient, Aphrodisiac, Carminative, Diuretic, Emmenagogue, Expectorant, Nervine, Stimulant, Tonic.

Usage:
For kidney ailments and urinary infections. Also used for coughs and arthritis.

Dosage: 40 – 50 gms. Added to daily feed.

Warnings:
Parsley can act as a uterine stimulant and therefore should not be fed to pregnant mares.

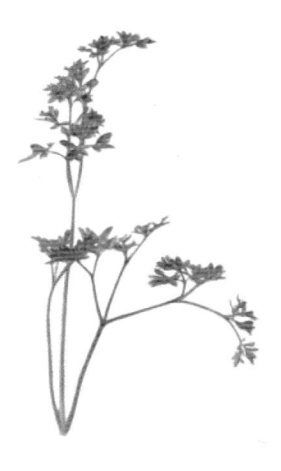

PERIWINKLE

Latin Name: Vinca major

Part Used: Aerial parts

Collection:
A native of Great Britain, Europe and the Orient. Springtime.

Actions:
Astringent, Diuretic, Haemostatic, Laxative, Nervine, Sedative, Tonic.

Usage:
Internally – Used for internal haemorrhaging, chronic diarrhoea, hormonal disorders, nose bleeds and mouth ulcers.

Externally – Suitable for use in a cream for soothing and healing inflammatory ailments of the skin and for bleeding piles.

Dosage: 20 – 30 gms. Added to daily feed.

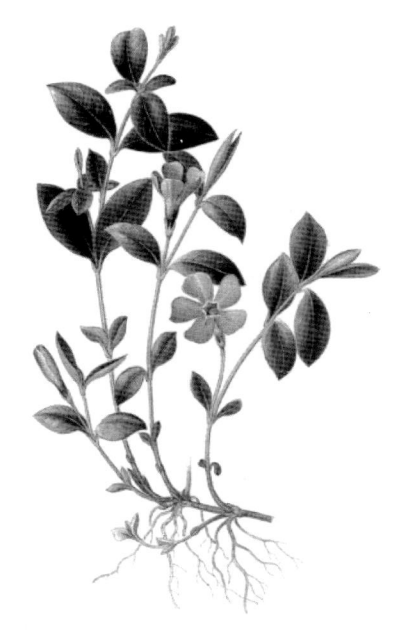

PSYLLIUM
Also known as Plantain

Latin Name: Plantago psyllium

Part Used: Seeds and leaves

Collection:
Grows throughout Southern Europe, Northern Africa and Southern Asia. Collect while flowering in summer.

Actions:
Astringent, Demulcent, Diuretic, Emollient, Expectorant, Laxative, Mucilage, Vulnerary.

Usage:
Psyllium seeds are said to be helpful in the prevention of sand colic.

Dosage: 40 – 50 gms. Added to daily feed.

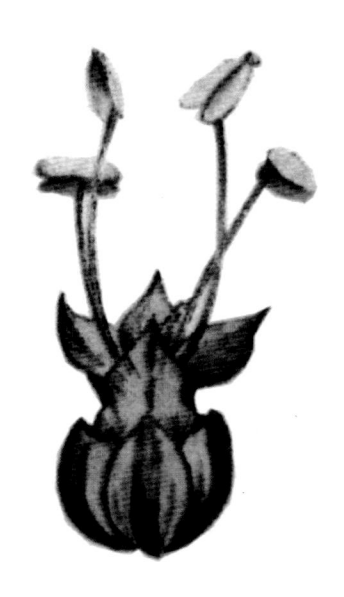

RASPBERRY

Latin Name: Rubus idaeus

Part Used: Leaves

Collection:
Grown throughout most of Europe and in some parts of Great Britain. Leaves can be collected throughout the growing season March to November.

Actions:
Alterative, Antispasmodic, Astringent, Cardiac, Diaphoretic, Diuretic, Emmenagogue, Febrifuge, Galactogogue, Haemostatic, Parturient, Stimulent, Stomachic, Tonic.

Usage:
A useful aid for the foaling mare. Ideally fed about one month before and after foaling. Tones pelvic and uterine muscles and enhances milk. Can also be helpful in the treatment of diarrhoea and mouth ulcers.

Combinations:
With Slippery Elm makes a good poultice for cleaning wounds.

Dosage: 40 – 50 gms. Added to daily feed.

Authors comments:
A very good herb to assist in foaling and cleansing although it is better not to feed it early in the pregnancy. We have also found it is often very effective in treating horses with diarrhoea – usually things improve within a few days.

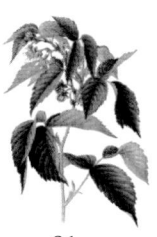

RED CLOVER
Also known as **Trefoil** and **Purple Clover**

Latin Name: Trifolium pratense

Part Used: Flowers

Collection:
Abundant in Britain, Europe and Northern Asia. Collected between May – September.

Actions:
Alterative, Antibiotic, Antifungal, Anti-inflammatory, Antimicrobial, Antispasmodic, Anti-tumour qualities, Antiviral, Astringent, Diaphoretic, Diuretic, Expectorant, Immune Stimulant, Laxative, Nervine, Restorative, Sedative, Stimulant, Tonic, Vulnerary.

Usage:
Internally – Used for coughs, diarrhoea and acts as a blood cleanser for skin problems such as mud fever. It also has calming and sedative qualities and can be helpful in the treatment for melanomas.

Externally - A compress can be used to treat rashes, ulcers, burns and sores.

Dosage: 30 – 40 gms. Added to daily feed.

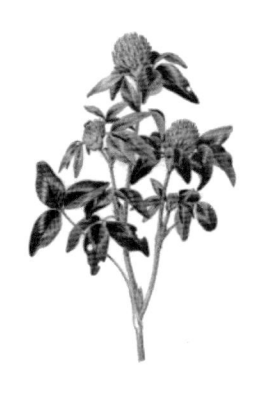

RED POPPY

Latin Name: Papaver rhoeas

Part Used: Petals and seeds

Collection:
Cultivated in Germany. The petals are collected in summer and autumn. Seeds collected in the autumn only.

Actions:
Analgesic, Anodyne, Demulcent, Hypnotic, Expectorant, Mucilage, Sedative, Tonic.

Usage:
Used for irritable coughs. It also has a soothing effect on the nervous system and it can be helpful for excitable horses.

Dosage: 15 – 20 gms. Added to daily feed.

Authors comments:
The seeds have a pleasant nutty flavour and are used sprinkled on bread.

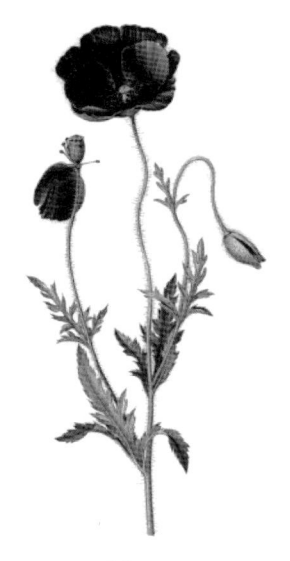

ROSEHIPS

Latin Name: Rosa canina

Part Used: Fruit and seeds

Collection:
Grows in Europe. Rosehips are the commonest of English wild roses but they are not as plentiful in Scotland. The fruit is collected late summer.

Actions:
Antimicrobial, Antipyretic, Antiseptic, Antispasmodic, Aperient, Astringent, Mild diuretic, Mucilage, Stomachic, Tonic.

Usage:
To promote hoof growth. Can be fed for exhaustion, constipation and as an aid to prevent scouring.

Dosage: 30 – 40 gms. Added to daily feed.

Authors comments:
The high levels of vitamin C (up to 1%) help the bodies natural defences. Rosehips have been shown to be a good natural supplement to promote hoof growth.

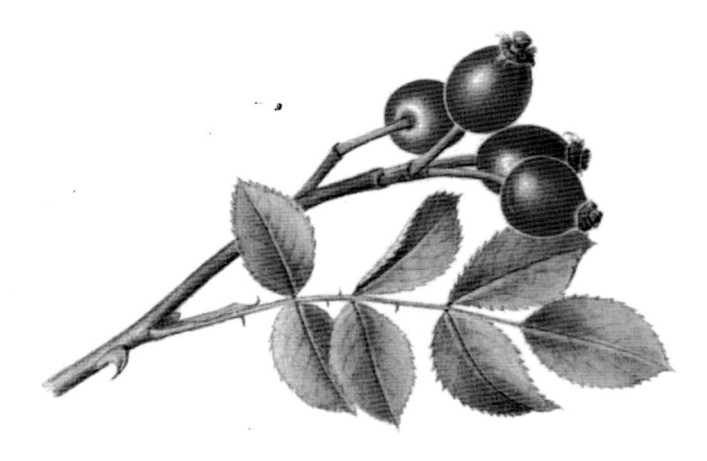

Rosehips
Rosa canina

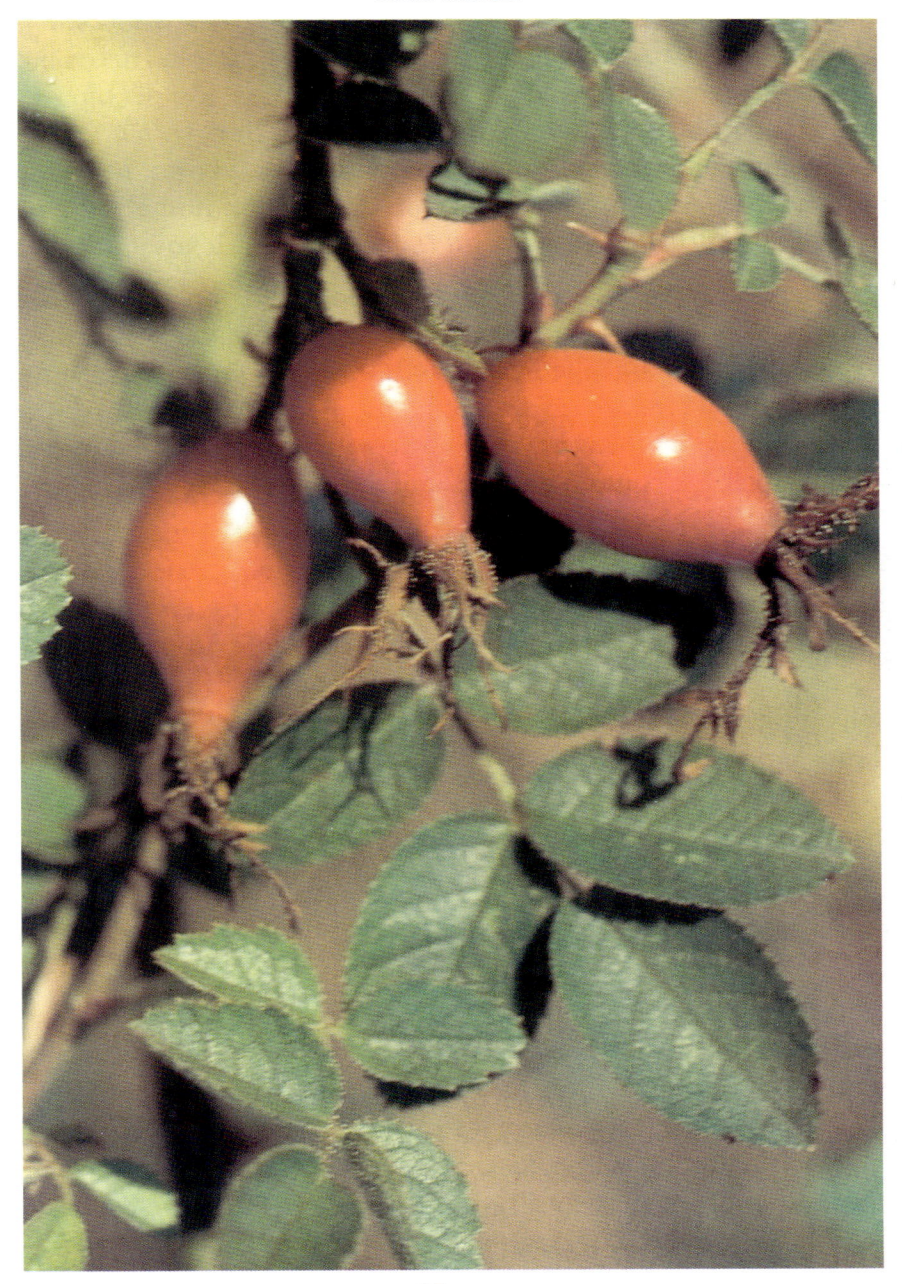

ROSEMARY

Latin Name: Rosmarinus officinalis

Part used: Leaves and young shoots

Collection:
Native to the Mediterranean region. Mostly imported from Spain, France and Morocco. Can be collected whilst flowering in summer.

Actions:
Anodyne, Analgesic, Antidepressant, Anti-inflammatory, Antipyretic, Antirheumatic, Antiseptic, Antispasmodic, Aperient, Aromatic, Astringent, Carminative, Cholagogue, Diaphoretic, Diuretic, Emmenagogue, Nervine, Rubefacient, Sedative, Stimulant, Stomachic, Tonic.

Usage:
Circulatory and nervine stimulant, digestion, rheumatism, diarrhoea.

Dosage: 20 – 30 gms. Added to daily feed.

Warnings:
Essential oil can be detectable in blood tests.

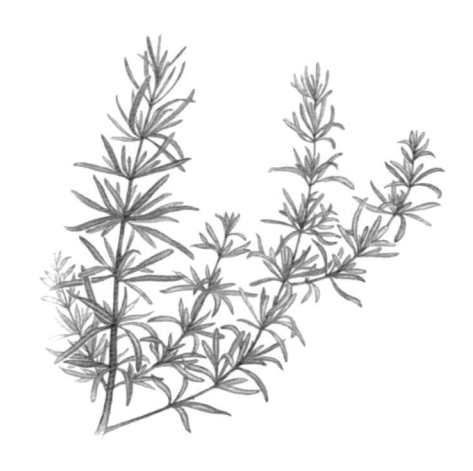

Rosemary
Rosmarinus officinalis

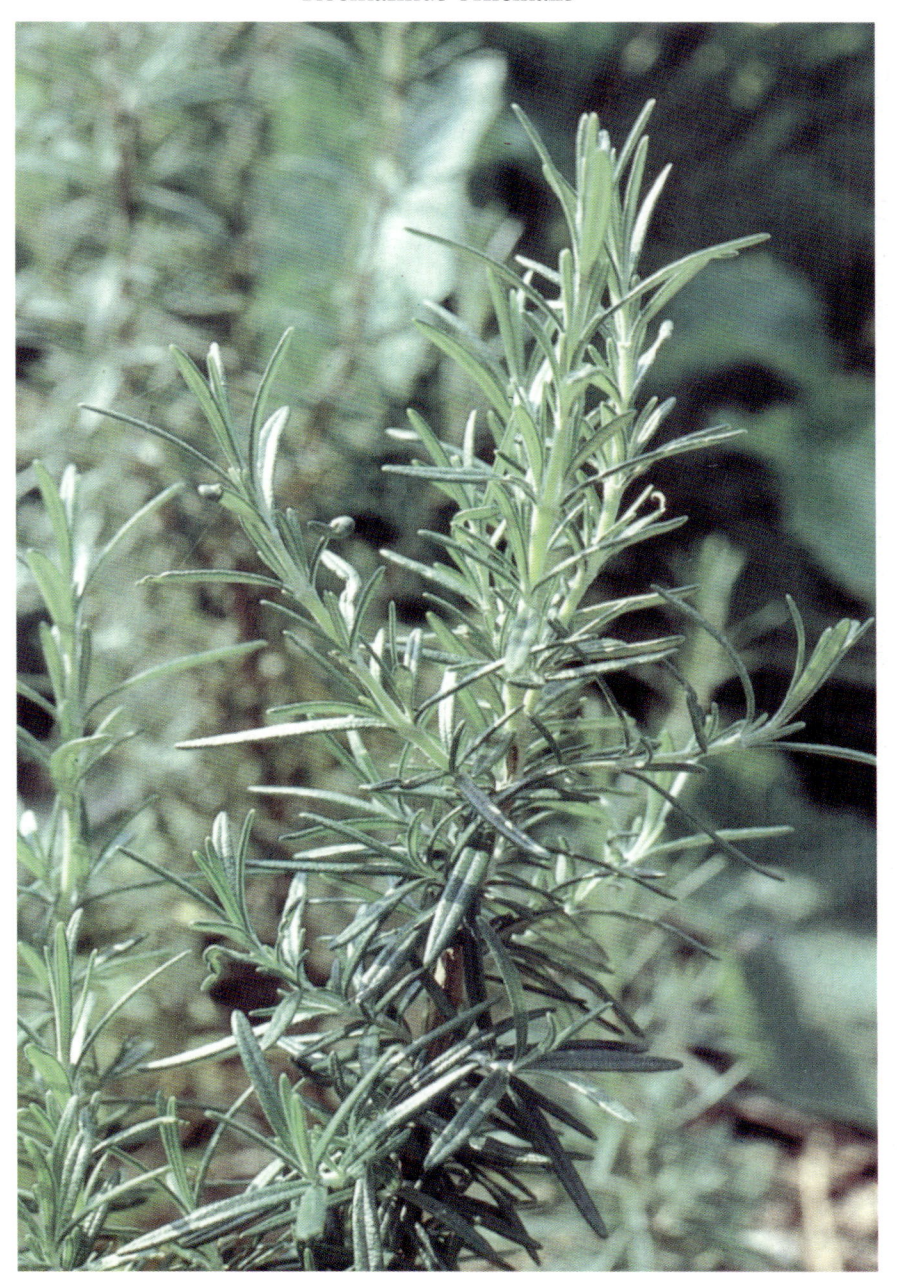

SAGE
Also known as **Red Sage**

Latin Name: Salvia officinalis

Part used: Leaves

Collection:
Native to the Mediterranean but cultivated elsewhere in Europe. It is grown commercially in Central and Southern England and harvested during June and July.

Actions:
Alterative, Antifungal, Antigalactagogue, Antimicrobial, Antipyretic, Antiseptic, Antispasmodic, Aromatic, Astringent, Carminative, Diuretic, Emmenagogue, Febrifuge, Nervine, Spasmolytic, Stimulant, Tonic, Vulnerary.

Usage:
Reduces sweating and lactation. Good for coughs, colds and nervous conditions. Also used for gastrointestinal disorders, wind colic and mouth infections.

Dosage: 20 – 30 gms. Added to daily feed.

Warning:
Do not feed to pregnant mares.

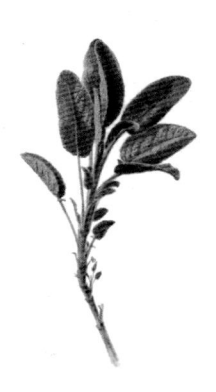

Sage
Salvia officinalis

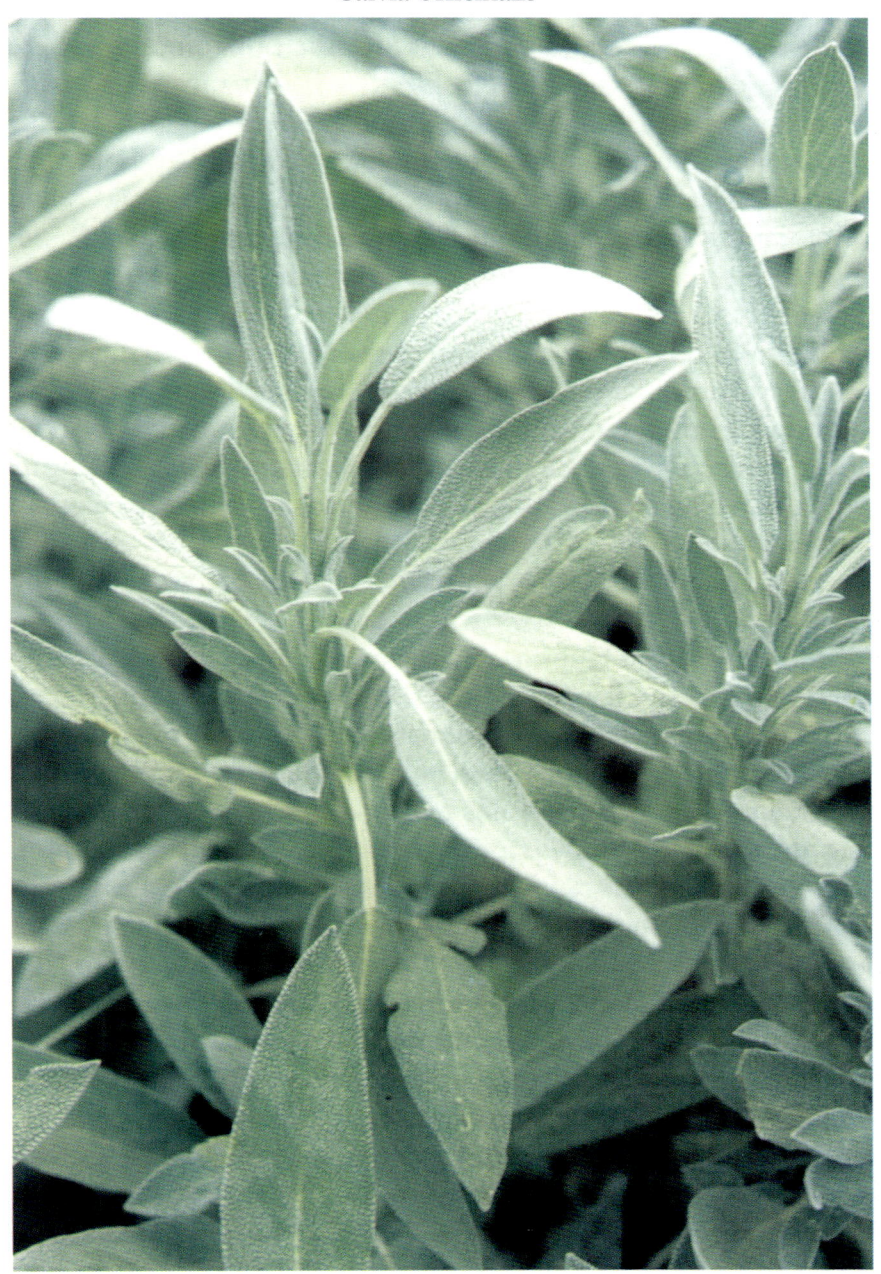

SAW PALMETTO

Latin Name: Serenoa serrulata

Part Used: Berries

Collection:
Thrives in the warm climates of Southern California to Florida. Gathered between September and January.

Actions:
Anti-Inflammatory, Antigalactagogue, Antiseptic, Antispasmodic, Aphrodisiac, Astringent, Diuretic, Expectorant, Nervine, Sedative, Stimulant, Tonic.

Usage:
For respiratory disorders, coughs and colds. It is said to boost male sex hormones.

Dosage: 15 – 20 gms. Added to daily feed.

SLIPPERY ELM

Latin Name: Ulmus fulva

Part Used: Inner bark

Collection:
A small tree abundant in various parts of North America. It is recommended that 10 year old bark is used. Harvested in spring.

Actions:
Anti-inflammatory, Antiseptic, Astringent, Demulcent, Diuretic, Emollient, Expectorant, Mucilage, Pectoral, Tonic, Vulnerary.

Usage:
Internally – An aid for digestion, diarrhoea and bronchial problems

Externally – For ulcers and abscesses.

Combinations:
Can be mixed with Marshmallow for digestive problems.

Dosage: 15 – 20 gms. Added to daily feed.

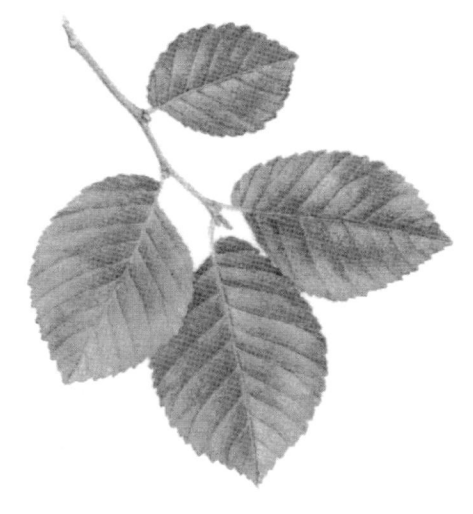

ST JOHNS WORT

Latin Name: Hypericum perforatum

Part used: Flowers and leaves

Collection:
Common throughout Europe including Britain. Collected when in flower.

Actions:
Alterative, Analgesic, Antibacterial, Antidepressant, Antifungal, Anti-inflammatory, Antispasmodic, Antiseptic, Antiviral, Aromatic, Astringent, Cholagogue, Diuretic, Emmenagogue, Expectorant, Sedative, Nervine, Vulnerary.

Usage:
For inflammation of the internal organs, disorders of the female reproductive system, rheumatic pain, stress, anxiety and tension. An effective sedative.

Dosage: 15 – 20 gms. Added to daily feed.

Warning:
Not recommended for long term use. Can make fair skinned horses especially sensitive to sun (photosensitivity).

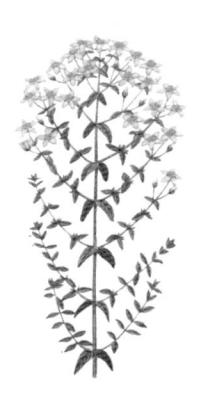

St Johns Wort
Hypericum perforatum

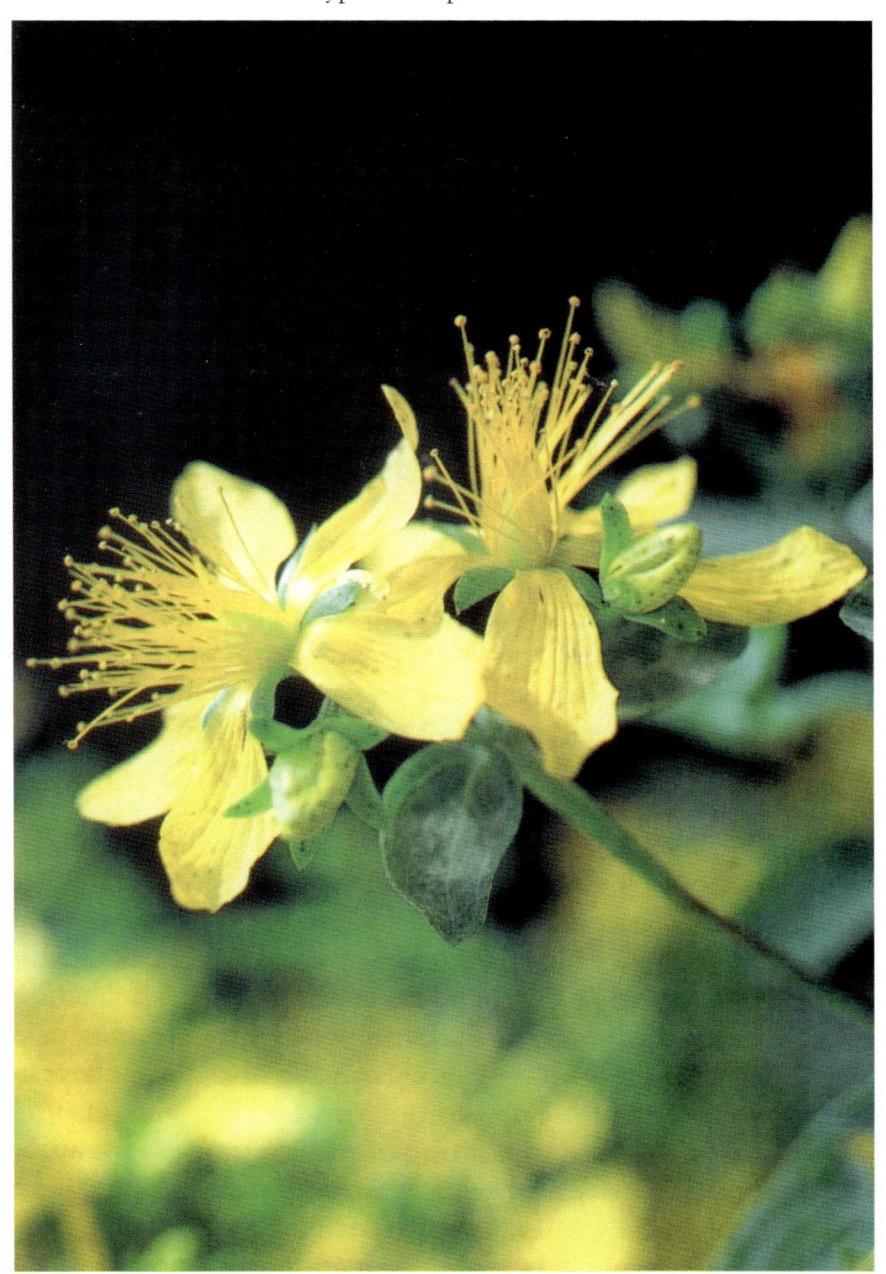

STRAWBERRY

Latin Name: Fragaria vesca

Part Used: Leaves

Collection:
Grows throughout the Northern Hemisphere. Collected during Summer.

Actions:
Alterative, Antiseptic, Aromatic, Astringent, Bitter, Diuretic, Laxative, Tonic.

Usage:
Used to treat fevers and for kidney and urinary disease. Also helpful in cases of diarrhoea and anaemia.

Dosage: 20 – 30 gms. Added to daily feed.

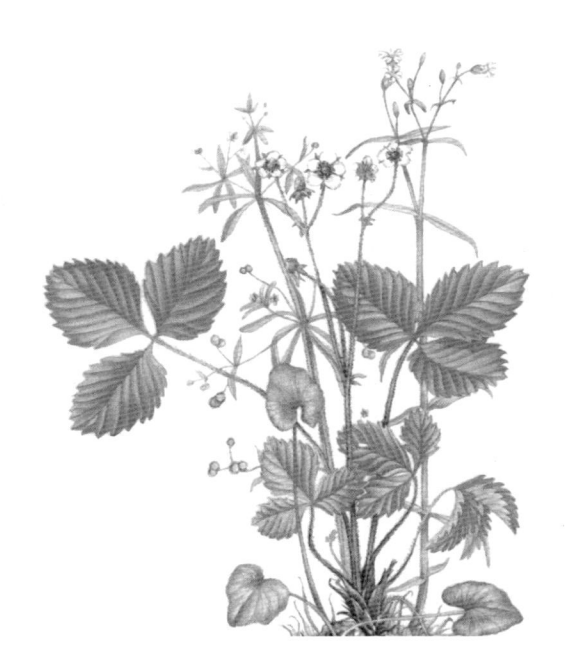

TEA TREE

Also known as **Cajeput** and **White Tea Tree**

Latin Name: Melaleuca leucadendron

Part Used: Oil

Collection:
Habitat East India, Tropical Australia. The oil is distilled from the fresh leaves and stalks.

Actions:
Antiseptic, Anti-Fungal, Anthelmintic, Diaphoretic.

Usage:
The diluted oil is usually applied externally for conditions of the skin. Good for sweet itch, burns and fungal infections such as ringworm

Authors comments:
Recommended for external use only.

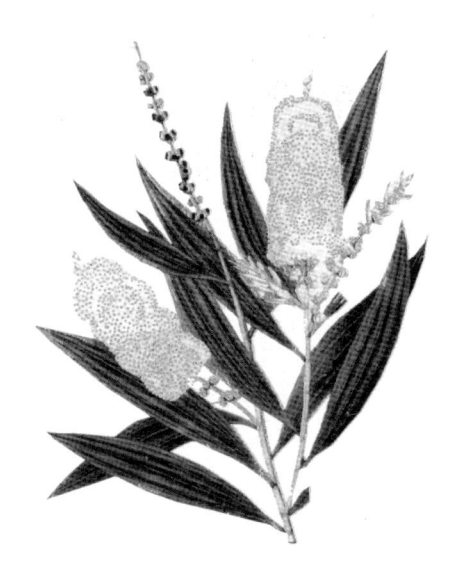

THYME

Latin Name: Thymus vulgaris

Part Used: Leaves and Flowering Tops.

Collection:
It is cultivated in most countries with temperate climates. Garden Thyme is an improved cultivated form of Wild Thyme. Harvested between June and August.

Actions:
Anthelmintic, Anticatarrhal, Antifungal, Antimicrobial, Antiseptic, Antispasmodic, Aromatic, Astringent, Carminative, Diaphoretic, Emmenagogue, Expectorant, Febrifuge, Nervine, Rubefacient, Sedative, Stimulant, Tonic, Vulnerary.

Usage:
Internally – Used for respiratory ailments, coughs, sore throats, digestive problems and indigestion or wind colic.

Externally – Can be used as an ointment for swellings and warts.

Dosage: 30 – 40 gms. Added to daily feed.

Authors comments: Reputed to be "A strengthener of the lungs".

Warning: Avoid feeding large amounts to pregnant mares.

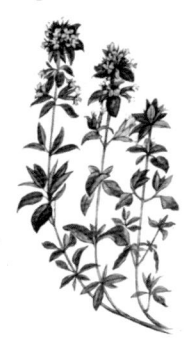

Thyme
Thymus vulgaris

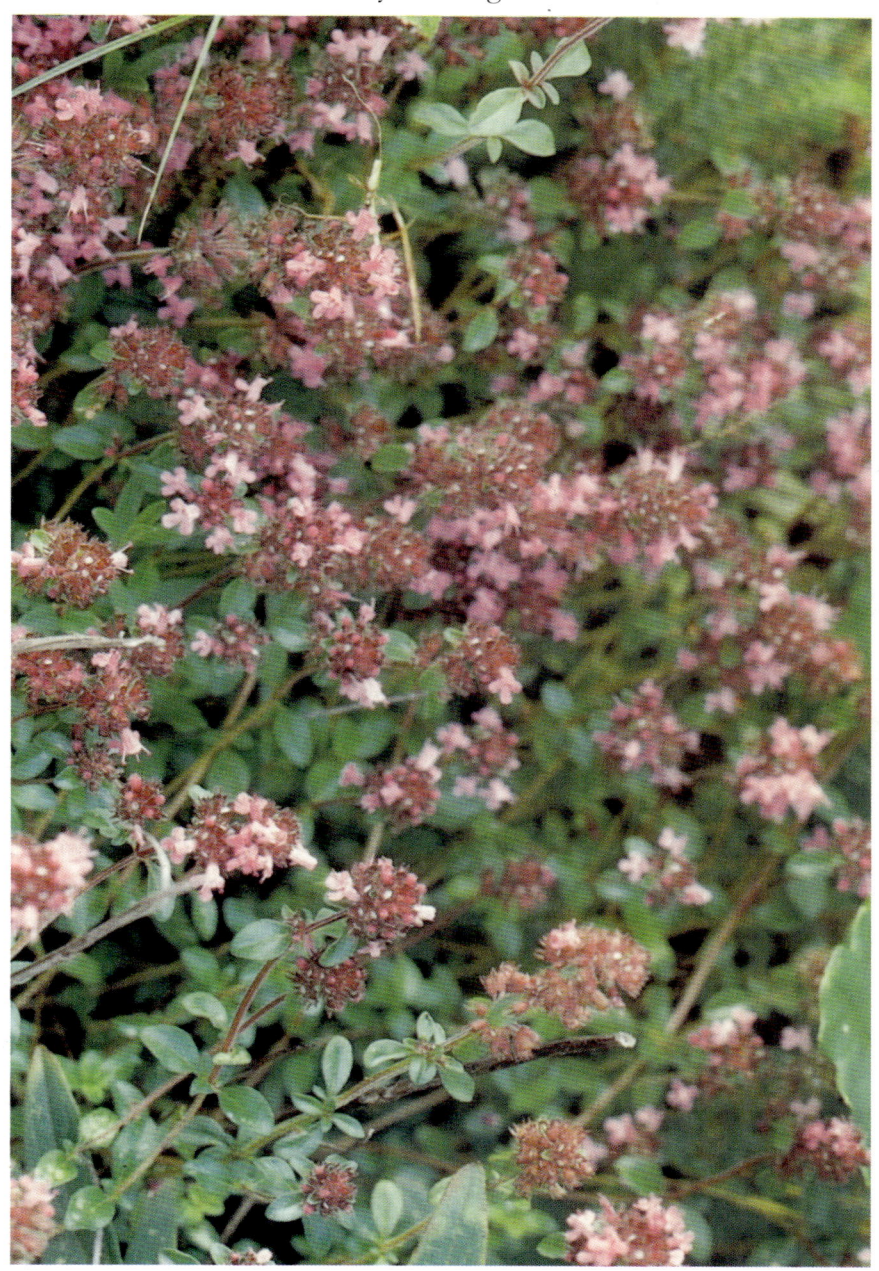

VALERIAN

Latin Name: Valeriana officinalis

Part Used: Root

Collection:
Available in Europe and Northern Asia. Roots of at least two years old should be collected during late Autumn.

Actions:
Analgesic, Anodyne, Antispasmodic, Aromatic, Bitter, Carminative, Diuretic, Febrifuge, Hypnotic, Laxative, Nervine, Sedative, Stimulant, Tonic, Vermifuge.

Usage:
Calms and relaxes. It is good for nervous over excitable horses and for stressful or anxious situations. Can be helpful in settling the digestive system.

Combinations:
Combines well with other relaxing herbs, such as Chamomile and Hops to make a general calming blend.

Dosage: 30 – 40 gms. Added to daily feed.

Authors Comments:
Regarded as a non addictive herb without side effects. Does not adversely affect performance in competition.

Warnings:
It has been stated that some governing bodies are testing for the use of Valerian Root during competitions. Although it has been in regular use world wide for a number of years, at the time of writing we are not aware of any test resulting in the disqualification of any competitor to date. For those concerned about competitions in the U.S.A. there are other calming herbs that can be used as an alternative.

Valerian
Valeriana officinalis

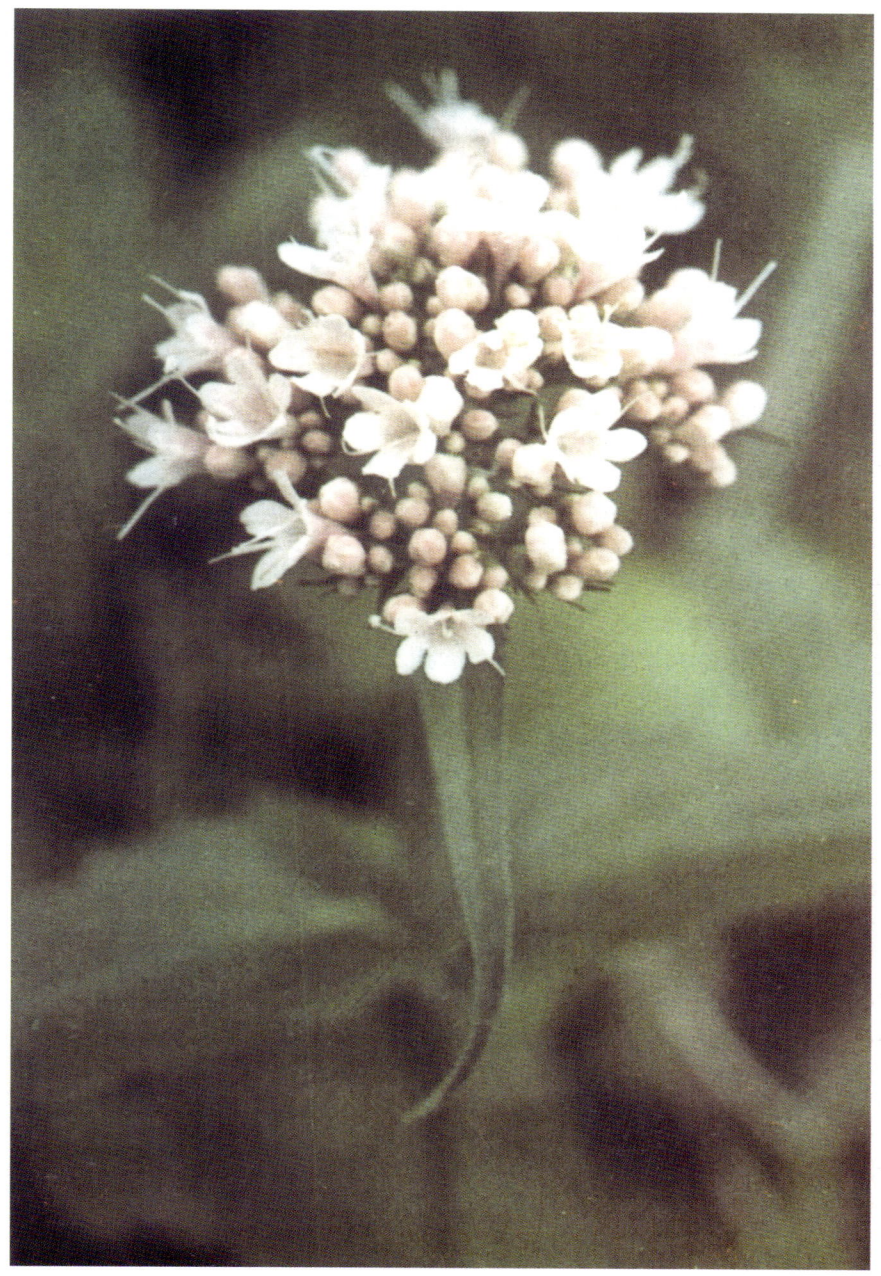

VERVAIN

Latin Name: Verbena officinalis

Part Used: Leaves and flowering heads

Collection:
Grown throughout Europe, China and Japan. Collect just before flowers open in July.

Actions:
Alterative, Antidepressant, Antispasmodic, Astringent, Bitter, Cholagogue, Diaphoretic, Emmenagogue, Expectorant, Febrifuge, Galactogogue, Hepatic, Mucilage, Nervine, Pectoral, Sedative, Stimulant, Tonic.

Usage:
A very good herb that can be used for a number of conditions including fevers, ulcers, tension, stress, nervous disorders and liver complaints.

Dosage: 40 – 50 gms. Added to daily feed.

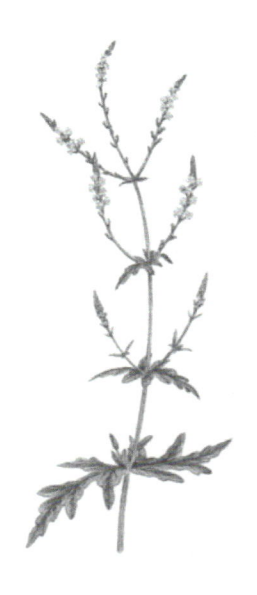

WILLOW (WHITE)

Latin Name: Salix alba

Part Used: Bark

Collection:
Thrives in the favoured climate of Central and Southern Europe. The bark is easily separated through the summer.

Actions:
Alterative, Analgesic, Anodyne, Anti-inflammatory, Antipyretic, Antiseptic, Antispasmodic, Astringent, Bitter, Diaphoretic, Diuretic, Febrifuge, Tonic, Vermifuge.

Usage:
Contains tannins which are very good for the digestive system. The salicin reduces inflammation and relieves pain. Good for rheumatism, arthritis and in reducing fevers.

Dosage: 30 - 40 gms. Added to daily feed.

Authors comments:
The characteristics of White Willow are very similar to Aspirin, which is a chemical substitute for salicin. White Willow naturally contains salicin which is also present in Meadowsweet.

Warnings:
Since White Willow is in effect "a natural form of Aspirin" it could be regarded as a prohibitive substance for competition purposes. It should also not be used long term for pregnant mares.

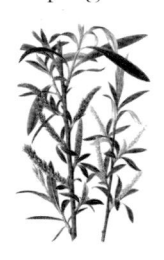

WITCH HAZEL

Also known as **Spotted Alder, Winterbloom.**

Latin Name: Hamamelis virginiana

Part Used: Bark and leaves

Collection:
Grows in the Eastern United States of America and Canada. Leaves are gathered in the summer. The bark is gathered in the spring.

Actions:
Anti-inflammatory, Antiseptic, Astringent, Bitter, Haemostatic, Sedative, Tonic, Vulnerary.

Usage:
Internally - It is used for haemorrhaging from the lungs and for stomach intestinal ulcers and diarrhoea.

Externally - Ideal for use as a tincture or cream for bruises and inflammatory swellings, bites and burns. Also useful for the treatment of piles in foals.

Authors comments:
Use only externally unless under veterinary supervision.

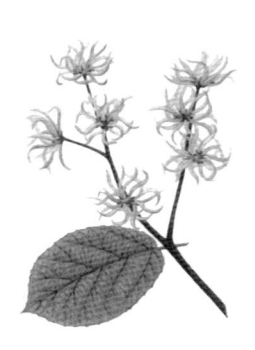

WORMWOOD
Also known as **Green Ginger**

Latin Name: Artemisia absinthium

Part Used: Whole herb

Collection:
Grows throughout the world including Europe, Siberia and the United States of America. Leaves and tops gathered in July and August when the plant is in flower and dried.

Actions:
Anthelmintic, Anti-inflammatory, Antiseptic, Antispasmodic, Aromatic, Bitter, Carminative, Cholagogue, Diaphoretic, Diuretic, Emmenagogue, Febrifuge, Haemostatic, Hepatic, Stimulant, Stomachic, Tonic, Vermifuge.

Usage:
To help prevent worms and for digestion and appetite.

Dosage: 15 – 20 gms. Added to daily feed.

Warning: Do not feed to pregnant mares.

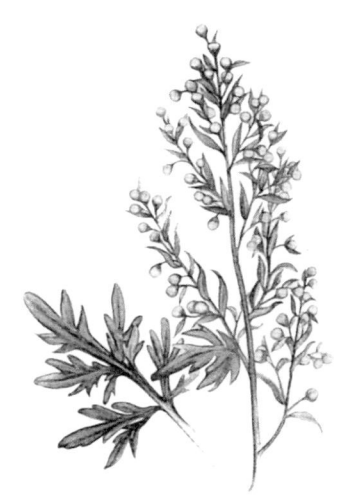

YARROW

Latin Name: Achillea millefolium

Part Used: The whole plant; stems, leaves and flowers

Collection:
A very hardy plant that will almost grow anywhere in meadows and can become a troublesome weed. Collected whilst in flower in August.

Actions:
Alterative, Antibacterial, Anticatarrhal, Anti-inflammatory, Antipyretic, Antiseptic, Antispasmodic, Aromatic, Astringent, Carminative, Diaphoretic, Diuretic, Emmenagogue, Febrifuge, Haemostatic, Hepatic, Stimulant, Stomachic, Tonic, Vulnerary.

Usage:
For digestion, appetite, fevers, kidney disorders and urinary infections.

Dosage: 30 – 40 gms. Added to daily feed.

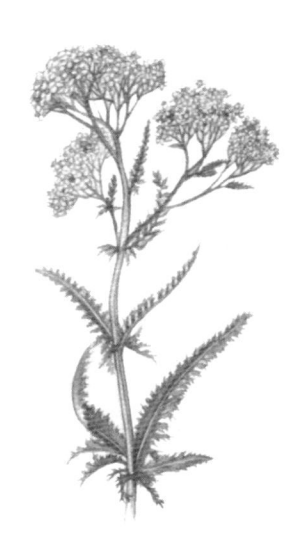

Yarrow
Achillea millefolium

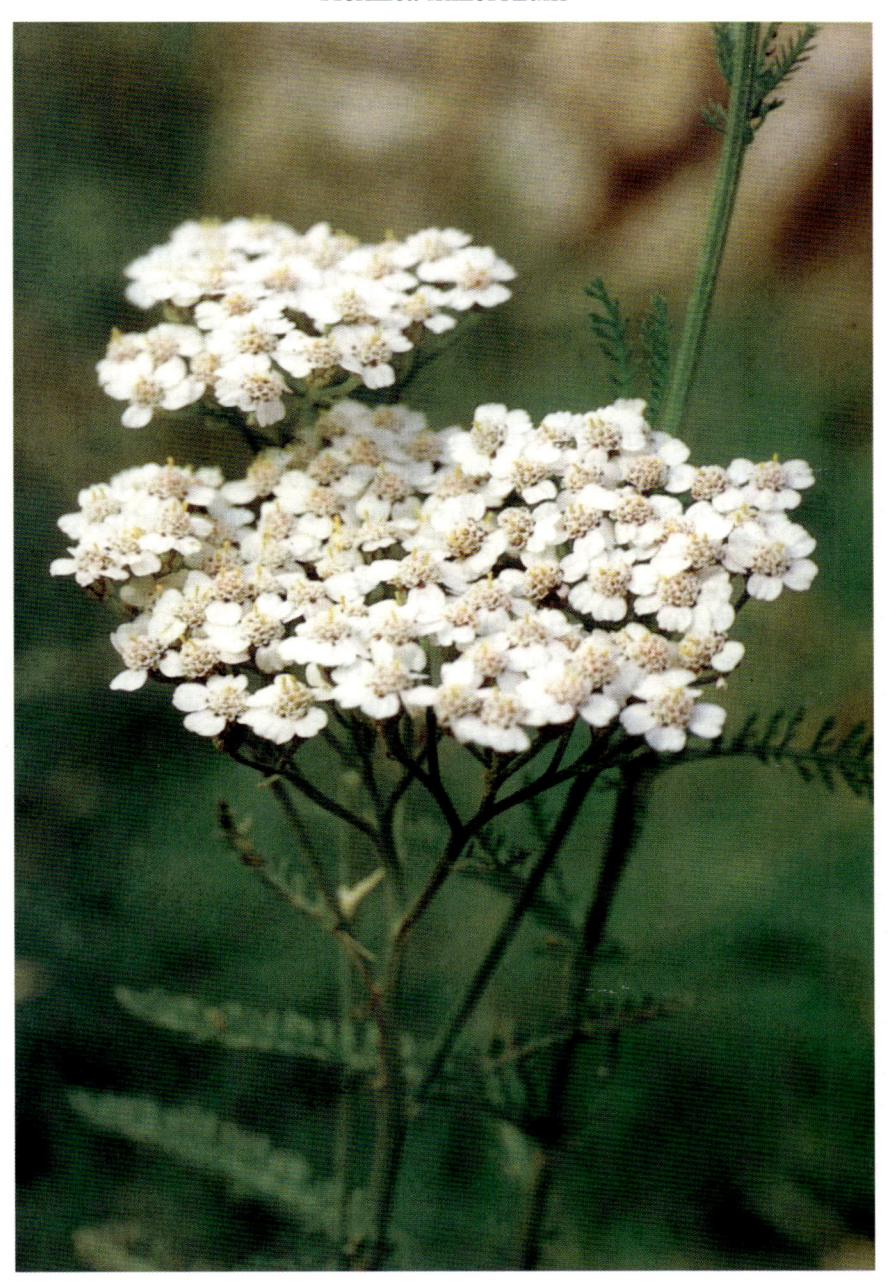

SECTION THREE

Herb Actions	109
Vitamins and Minerals	119
Other Herbal Preparations	127
Aromatherapy	129
Homeopathy	131
Bach Flower Remedies	132
McTimoney Chiropractic	133

HERB ACTIONS

Acrid
Hot to taste. Can cause heat and irritation when applied to skin.
Buckwheat.

Alterative
These are herbs that will help restore the correct function of the body towards good health and well being. Also known as 'blood cleansers'.
Alfalfa, Bladderwrack, Burdock, Celery, Chamomile, Cleavers, Dandelion, Echinacea, Garlic, Lime Tree, Liquorice, Marigold, Marjoram, Meadowsweet, Mint, Nettles, Raspberry, Red Clover, Sage, St Johns Wort, Strawberry, Vervain, Willow, Yarrow.

Analgesic
Analgesics are herbs that reduce pain.
Chamomile, Devils Claw, Hops, Marigold, Mint, Red Poppy, Rosemary, St Johns Wort, Valerian, Willow.

Anodyne
Reduces pain and irritation.
Chamomile, Devils Claw, Hops, Mint, Red Poppy, Rosemary, Valerian, Willow.

Antacid
Neutralizes acidity in gut.
Meadowsweet.

Anthelmintic
Anthelmintics cause the destruction and expulsion of worms from the digestive system. The following are still available:
Alfalfa, Aloe, Garlic, Tea Tree, Thyme, Wormwood.

Antibacterial (Antibiotic)
To destroy or stop the growth of bacterial infections.
Basil, Echinacea, Liquorice, Marigold, Mint, St Johns Wort, Yarrow.

Antibiotic
Substances used to destroy bacteria and other disease causing organisms with the action of helping to withstand infection or infestation.
Bladderwrack, Couch Grass, Echinacea, Garlic, Red Clover.
Also Cider Apple Vinegar has antibiotic qualities.

Anticatarrhal
Anticatarrhal herbs help in the removal of excess catarrh.
Coltsfoot, Echinacea, Eyebright, Garlic, Golden Rod, Mint, Thyme, Yarrow.

Antidepressant
Alleviates depression.
Damiana, Lavender, Marigold, Rosemary, St Johns Wort, Vervain.

Antifungal
To kill or reduce fungal infections.
Basil, Ginkgo, Golden Rod, Marigold, Red Clover, Sage, St Johns Wort, Tea Tree, Thyme.

Antigalactagogue
Will prevent or reduce the secretion of milk.
Sage, Saw Palmetto.

Antihistamine
Has the action of reducing the body's release of histamine.
Buckwheat, Garlic, Parsley.

Antihypothyroid
Having an action to stimulate thyroid function.
Bladderwrack.

Anti-inflammatory
Anti-inflammatory herbs help reduce inflammation. Some are used externally only.
Arnica, Celery, Chamomile, Comfrey, Devils Claw, Echinacea, Eyebright, Golden Rod, Lime Tree, Liquorice, Marigold, Meadowsweet, Mint, Red Clover, Rosemary, Saw Palmetto, Slippery Elm, St Johns Wort, Willow, Witch Hazel, Wormwood, Yarrow.

Antilithic
To help prevent the formation of stones in the urinary system. They can also help in expelling them from the body.
Couch Grass.

Antimicrobial
Anti-microbial herbs help the body to destroy micro-organisms.
Burdock, Couch Grass, Echinacea, Garlic, Lavender, Marigold, Mint, Red Clover, Rosehips, Sage, Thyme.

Antipyretic
A Febrifuge. An agent that reduces fever.
Meadowsweet, Rosehips, Rosemary, Sage, Willow, Yarrow.

Antirheumatic
Helps in the prevention or relief of rheumatism.
Bladderwrack, Dandelion, Devils Claw, Meadowsweet, Parsley, Rosemary.

Antiseptic
Combats and neutralizes bacteria, and prevents infection.
Aniseed, Burdock, Celery, Chamomile, Cleavers, Echinacea, Eyebright, Fennel, Garlic, Golden Rod, Hops, Lavender, Marigold, Marjoram, Meadowsweet, Mint, Nettle, Parsley, Rosehips, Rosemary, Sage, Saw Palmetto, Slippery Elm, St Johns Wort, Strawberry, Tea Tree, Thyme, Willow, Witch Hazel, Wormwood, Yarrow.

Antispasmodic
To prevent or ease spasms or cramps in the body.
Aniseed, Balm, Basil, Chamomile, Cleavers, Fennel, Garlic, Golden Rod, Hawthorn, Hops, Horehound, Lavender, Lime Tree, Liquorice, Marigold, Marjoram, Meadowsweet, Mint, Parsley, Raspberry, Red Clover, Rosehips, Rosemary, Sage, Saw Palmetto, St Johns Wort, Thyme, Valerian, Vervain, Willow, Wormwood, Yarrow.

Antiviral
To prevent or reduce viral infection.
Echinacea, Garlic, Liquorice, Mint, Red Clover, St Johns Wort.

Aperient
Mild laxatives.
Burdock, Cleavers, Couch Grass, Dandelion, Marigold, Parsley, Rosehips, Rosemary.

Aphrodisiac
To stimulate sexual desire and improve function.
Damiana, Echinacea, Fenugreek, Liquorice, Parsley, Saw Palmetto.

Appetizer
To stimulate and promote appetite.
Alfalfa, Fenugreek, Saw Palmetto.

Aromatic
Herbs that release a strong usually pleasant odour that can help to stimulate the digestive system.
Aniseed, Balm, Basil, Celery, Chamomile, Chaste Tree, Fennel, Fenugreek, Garlic, Golden Rod, Horehound, Marigold, Marjoram, Meadowsweet, Mint, Rosemary, Sage, St Johns Wort, Strawberry, Thyme, Valerian, Wormwood, Yarrow.

Astringent
Astringents contain tannins which help to bind and connect tissue and reduce discharges and secretions.
Buckwheat, Cleavers, Coltsfoot, Comfrey, Eyebright, Ginkgo, Golden Rod, Hawthorn, Hops, Horsetail, Lime Tree, Marigold, Marjoram, Marshmallow, Meadowsweet, Mint, Nettle, Periwinkle, Psyllium, Raspberry, Red Clover, Rosehips, Rosemary, Sage, Saw Palmetto, Slippery Elm, St Johns Wort, Strawberry, Thyme, Vervain, Willow, Witch Hazel, Yarrow.

Bitter
Bitter tasting herbs cause the taste buds to stimulate the digestive system.
Balm, Burdock, Celery, Chamomile, Coltsfoot, Damiana, Dandelion, Devils Claw, Eyebright, Ginkgo, Hops, Horehound, Marigold, Marjoram, Milk Thistle, Sage, Strawberry, Valerian, Vervain, Willow, Witch Hazel, Wormwood.

Cardiac Tonic
Cardiac tonics have a beneficial affect on the heart.
Hawthorn, Raspberry.

Calmative
Helps to gently calm nerves.
Balm, Chamomile, Marjoram, Mint.

Carminative
The carminative are rich in volatile oils that help relieve flatulence and settle the digestive system.
Aniseed, Balm, Basil, Celery, Chamomile, Chaste Tree, Fennel, Fenugreek, Garlic, Golden Rod, Horsetail, Lavender, Marjoram, Mint, Parsley, Rosemary, Sage, Thyme, Valerian, Wormwood, Yarrow.

Cholagogue
Cholagogues stimulate the release and secretion of bile into the intestine which can have a laxative effect on the digestive system.
Burdock, Dandelion, Garlic, Horehound, Lavender, Marigold, Milk Thistle, Rosemary, St Johns Wort, Vervain, Wormwood.

Demulcent
Demulcents contain mucilage that helps to soothe and protect internal tissue that has become inflamed.
Bladderwrack, Coltsfoot, Comfrey, Couch Grass, Fenugreek, Liquorice, Marshmallow, Milk Thistle, Psyllium, Red Poppy, Slippery Elm.

Diaphoretic
Diaphoretics promote sweating and can help in reducing fevers.
Balm, Burdock, Chamomile, Fenugreek, Garlic, Golden Rod, Horehound, Lime Blossom, Marigold, Marjoram, Mint, Raspberry, Red Clover, Rosemary, Tea Tree, Thyme, Vervain, Willow, Wormwood, Yarrow.

Diuretic
Diuretics increase the secretion of urine.
Alfalfa, Aniseed, Bladderwrack, Burdock, Celery, Cleavers, Coltsfoot, Couch Grass, Dandelion, Devils Claw, Fennel, Garlic, Golden Rod, Hawthorn, Hops, Horehound, Horsetail, Lavender, Lime Tree, Liquorice, Marigold, Marshmallow, Meadowsweet, Nettles, Parsley, Periwinkle, Psyllium, Raspberry, Red Clover, Rosehips, Rosemary, Sage, Saw Palmetto, Slippery Elm, St Johns Wort, Strawberry, Valerian, Willow, Wormwood, Yarrow.

Emmenagogue
Emmenagogues normalise and can act as a tonic to the female reproductive system. Some Emmenagogues can also have abortificient actions.
Aloe, Balm, Chamomile, Chaste Tree, Horehound, Horsetail, Marigold, Marjoram, Parsley, Raspberry, Rosemary, Sage, St Johns Wort, Thyme, Valerian, Vervain, Wormwood, Yarrow.

Emollient
For applying to the skin to soothe or protect it.
Bladderwrack, Coltsfoot, Comfrey, Fenugreek, Liquorice, Marshmallow, Psyllium, Slippery Elm.

Expectorant
Has the action of promoting the removal of excess amounts of mucus from the respiratory system.
Aniseed, Basil, Coltsfoot, Comfrey, Fennel, Fenugreek, Garlic, Ginkgo, Golden Rod, Horehound, Lime Tree, Liquorice, Marjoram, Marshmallow, Nettles, Parsley, Psyllium, Red Clover, Red Poppy, Saw Palmetto, Slippery Elm, St Johns Wort, Thyme, Vervain.

Febrifuge
Antipyretic. Helps the body to reduce fevers.
Balm, Garlic, Hops, Marigold, Mint, Raspberry, Sage, Thyme, Valerian, Vervain, Willow, Wormwood, Yarrow.

Galactogogue
Galactogogues help stimulate and increase the flow of mares milk.
Alfalfa, Aniseed, Basil, Fennel, Fenugreek, Horsetail, Marshmallow, Milk Thistle, Nettles, Raspberry, Vervain.

Haemostatic
To arrest bleeding and promote blood clotting.
Comfrey, Horsetail, Nettles, Periwinkle, Raspberry, Witch Hazel, Wormwood, Yarrow.

Hepatic
Helps strengthen the liver and increase the flow of bile.
Aloe, Celery, Dandelion, Fennel, Vervain, Wormwood, Yarrow.

Hypnotic
Hypnotics induce sleep.
Hops, Red Poppy, Valerian.

Immuno-stimulant
Enhances the body's immune system.
Echinacea, Red Clover.

Laxative
Promotes the evacuation of the bowels.
Aloe, Burdock, Cleavers, Couch Grass, Damiana, Dandelion, Fenugreek, Liquorice, Marshmallow, Periwinkle, Psyllium, Red Clover, Strawberry, Valerian.

Mucilage
Mucilaginous herbs contain gelatinous constituents that can be demulcent and emollient.
Bladderwrack, Burdock, Chamomile, Coltsfoot, Comfrey, Couch Grass, Fennel, Fenugreek, Garlic, Lime Tree, Marigold, Marshmallow, Meadowsweet, Psyllium, Red Poppy, Rosehips, Slippery Elm, Vervain.

Nervine
A nerve tonic that calms the nerves.
Alfalfa, Balm, Celery, Chamomile, Damiana, Eyebright, Ginkgo, Hops, Lavender, Lime Tree, Marjoram, Milk Thistle, Mint, Parsley, Periwinkle, Red Clover, Rosemary, Sage, Saw Palmetto, St Johns Wort, Thyme, Valerian, Vervain.

Parturient
Stimulates uterine contractions to induce and assist foaling.
Raspberry.

Pectoral
Pectoral herbs help to strengthen and heal the respiratory system.
Aniseed, Coltsfoot, Comfrey, Garlic, Horehound, Liquorice, Marshmallow, Slippery Elm, Vervain.

Relaxant
Relaxes nerves and muscles; relieves tension.
Lavender, Liquorice.

Restorative
Helps restore health and strength.
Chaste Tree, Fenugreek, Red Clover.

Rubefacient
When rubefacients are applied to the skin they cause a gentle local irritation and stimulate the dilation of the capillaries, thus increasing circulation in the skin. The blood is drawn from deeper parts of the body into the skin and thus often internal pains are relieved.
Fennel, Garlic, Lavender, Marjoram, Mint, Nettle, Rosemary, Thyme.

Sedative
Sedatives calm the nervous system, reduce stress and nervousness and induce sleep.
Balm, Basil, Bladderwrack, Celery, Chamomile, Chaste Tree,
Devils Claw, Ginkgo, Hawthorn, Hops, Horehound, Lavender, Mint, Periwinkle, Red Clover, Red Poppy, Rosemary, Saw Palmetto,
St. Johns Wort, Thyme, Valerian, Vervain, Witch Hazel.

Spasmolytic
Spasmolytics reduce spasms of the intestines and bronchials.
Sage.

Stimulant
A stimulant acts to enliven the physiological function of the body.
Aniseed, Arnica, Bladderwrack, Celery, Damiana, Dandelion, Fennel, Garlic, Golden Rod, Hops, Horehound, Lavender, Marigold, Marjoram, Milk Thistle, Mint, Nettle, Parsley, Raspberry, Red Clover, Rosemary, Sage, Saw Palmetto, Thyme, Valerian, Vervain, Wormwood, Yarrow.

Stomachic
Helps to strengthen stomach function.
Aniseed, Balm, Basil, Celery, Chamomile, Dandelion, Eyebright, Fennel, Fenugreek, Hops, Horehound, Lavender, Liquorice, Marjoram, Meadowsweet, Mint, Raspberry, Rosehips, Rosemary, Wormwood, Yarrow.

Tonic
Tonic herbs strengthen and invigorate a specific organ system or the whole body.
Alfalfa, Aniseed, Balm, Bladderwrack, Burdock, Celery, Chamomile, Chaste Tree, Cleavers, Coltsfoot, Comfrey, Couch Grass, Damiana, Dandelion, Echinacea, Eyebright, Fennel, Fenugreek, Garlic, Hawthorn, Hops, Horehound, Lavender, Lime Tree, Liquorice, Marigold, Marjoram, Marshmallow, Meadowsweet, Milk Thistle, Mint, Nettle, Parsley, Periwinkle, Raspberry, Red Clover, Red Poppy, Rosehips, Rosemary, Sage, Saw Palmetto, Slippery Elm, Strawberry, Thyme, Valerian, Vervain, Willow, Witch Hazel, Wormwood, Yarrow.

Vermifuge
Expels or repels intestinal worms.
Alfalfa, Aloe, Couch Grass, Garlic, Hops, Marigold, Valerian, Willow, Wormwood.

Vulnerary
Vulneraries are applied externally to aid the body in the healing of wounds.
Aloe, Arnica, Burdock, Chamomile, Cleavers, Comfrey, Fenugreek, Garlic, Golden Rod, Horehound, Horsetail, Marigold, Marshmallow, Psyllium, Red Clover, Sage, Slippery Elm, St Johns Wort, Thyme, Witch Hazel, Yarrow.

VITAMINS & MINERALS

All horses have vitamin and mineral requirements that ideally would form part of their normal well balanced diet.

In looking at the requirements for a horse it is necessary to consider the nutritional requirements as a whole in relation to the age, size and type of the horse together with the level of physical activity. When considering vitamin and mineral supplementation the advice of a qualified equine nutritionist is invaluable. Most feed companies offer the services of a nutritionist and they are only too pleased to advise on any supplementation requirements you may have, whilst taking into account the existing diet and conditions.

There is a tendency by some horse owners to over supplement their horse. The horse may be receiving a good balanced feedstuff containing all necessary vitamins and minerals but still several other synthetic products are added in the belief that these will help the horse. In many cases these supplements are at best wasted and in others they can actually work against the principle of an ideal balanced diet.

There are now so many synthetically produced vitamins and minerals available to herbivores. Many are even promoted as natural supplements. However there is nothing more natural to the horses system than herbs. If fed correctly they will benefit the horse, but where they are not required they will simply pass through, avoiding the chemical build ups that can result from some supplements.

The following is a brief guide to vitamins, minerals and trace elements that are included in a horses diet together with a brief description of their function. Also listed are some common herbs that include these substances. This guide is an indication only of some of the qualities and characteristics of some common herbs. As always the advice is to consult an equine nutritionist to establish the correct balance of vitamins and minerals for your horse. Also remember that herbs can have many functions therefore you should check with a herbalist before mixing several together.

SOME VITAMINS, MINERAL AND TRACE ELEMENT PROPERTIES IN HERBS

Minerals

Calcium (Ca)
Calcium is essential for the growth, maintenance and development of bone, teeth and hooves. It is also involved in blood coagulation, lactation and nerve and muscle function.
Alfalfa, Bladderwrack, Buckwheat, Chamomile, Cleavers, Coltsfoot, Comfrey, Dandelion, Fenugreek, Garlic, Hops, Horsetail, Liquorice, Marshmallow, Meadowsweet, Nettles, Parsley, Red Clover, Rosehips, Slippery Elm, Willow, Yarrow.

Phosphorus (P)
Phosphorus is closely related to calcium in maintaining the bony structure. It promotes eyesight and helps maintain the brain and nerve coordination.
Aniseed, Bladderwrack, Buckwheat, Dandelion, Fenugreek, Garlic, Golden Rod, Lime Tree, Liquorice, Marigold, Meadowsweet, Nettles, Parsley, Rosehips, Yarrow.

Magnesium (Mg)
Magnesium is needed for normal cell metabolism and nerve and muscle function. It reduces excess acidity, calms the nerves and promotes health of the skin.
Alfalfa, Bladderwrack, Buckwheat, Dandelion, Hops, Marshmallow, Meadowsweet, Mint, Red Clover, Red Poppy, Slippery Elm.

Potassium (K)
Potassium is involved in body fluid regulation. It encourages healing of diseased tissues and stimulates the liver. Grass and hay usually contain high levels of potassium.
Alfalfa, Bladderwrack, Buckwheat, Chamomile, Cider Apple Vinegar, Coltsfoot, Comfrey, Couchgrass, Dandelion, Eyebright, Fennel, Garlic, Horsetail, Liquorice, Meadowsweet, Mint, Nettle, Parsley, Wormwood.

Sodium (Na)
Like potassium, sodium is involved in body fluid regulation. It is also involved in the absorption of sugars and amino acids from the gut. It helps prevent disease of mucus membranes and maintains the health of the urinary system. A salt block in the stable will allow free choice access to sodium.
Bladderwrack, Cleavers, Comfrey, Dandelion, Fennel, Garlic, Marshmallow, Meadowsweet, Nettle, Red Clover.

Trace elements

Copper (Cu)
Copper is involved in the formation of bone, cartilage, hair pigment and in the utilisation of iron in the production of red blood cells. There appears to be a relationship between low copper levels and poor performance in competition horses.
Burdock, Cleavers, Dandelion, Fennel, Garlic, Parsley, Yarrow.

Zinc (Zn)
Zinc is involved in normal cell metabolism and is an enzyme activator. High levels of zinc can interfere with copper utilisation. A deficiency of zinc can result in skin problems, hair loss, scaly skin, poor wound healing and skeletal abnormalities.
Bladderwrack, Bran, Coltsfoot.

Manganese (Mn)
Manganese is involved in the process of cartilage formation. High calcium levels can reduce the absorption of manganese hence causing a deficiency. Manganese deficiency can affect bone development and reproduction. Levels of manganese in grass and hay can vary greatly.
Bladderwrack, Bran, Nettles, Oats.

Iron (Fe)
Iron is essential for red blood cell production, hence it helps in maintaining body resistance to disease and infection.
Signs of a deficiency can include lack of stamina and poor growth. A reduction in red cell production results in anaemia.
Alfalfa, Bladderwrack, Buckwheat, Burdock, Comfrey, Couch Grass, Dandelion,

Fenugreek, Garlic, Hawthorn, Hops, Nettles, Parsley, Periwinkle, Raspberry, Rosehips, Strawberry, Vervain, Wormwood.

Iodine (I)
Iodine has an effect on the production of hormones from the thyroid gland. Abnormal amounts can affect the oestrus cycle and hence the ability of a mare to conceive. It promotes the growth of hair.
Bladderwrack, Cleavers, Garlic, Marigold.

Selenium (Se)
Selenium is closely related to vitamin E. It is used for the maintanence of muscle tissue and a deficiency causes weak muscles and poor performance in racehorses. Excess selenium is toxic and can cause hair loss, stiff joints and anaemia. The normal requirement of selenium is not always available to horses grazing, although there are some areas where they have too high a level of selenium in the soil.
Linseed contains high levels of selenium as does *Garlic, Bladderwrack, Horsetail*.

Vitamins are divided into two groups; fat soluble and water soluble.

Fat soluble vitamins are found in green herbage and because they can be stored in the horses body the horse can retain enough of these vitamins in the summer to maintain the requirements throughout the year. However, horses that are stabled may require supplementary vitamins.

Water soluble vitamins are produced by micro-organisms in the horses gut therefore they do not need to be stored.

When a horse is fit and eating less forage the capacity of the hind gut is reduced. This results in less bacteria in the gut producing the vitamins, resulting in the need to supplement.

Water soluble vitamins

Vitamin B1 (Thiamin)
Thiamin helps regulate the release of energy from stored carbohydrates and a shortfall may show as a lack of energy or muscle weakness. Deficiency can result in a lack of appetite with subsequent loss of weight and weakness, impaired growth and in-coordination.
Dandelion, Rosehips.

Vitamin B2 (Riboflavin or Lactoflavin)
Riboflavin is important in protein and carbohydrate metabolism. A deficiency reduces energy and the bodies utilization of protein, thereby affecting condition and growth. Good quality grass and hay provide more than sufficient levels of Vitamin B2.
Dandelion, Rosehips.

Vitamin B3 (Niacin)
Niacin helps in the metabolism of carbohydrates, fats and proteins. A deficiency can lead to skin and digestive disorders. Signs of deficiency include a loss of appetite, reduction in growth and diarrhoea. The skin can become poor as the condition worsens.
Oil seeds contain vitamin B3.

Vitamin B12 (Cyanocobalamin)
Vitamin B12 is important for the production of red blood cells. A deficiency can result in loss of appetite and poor growth as well as anaemia due to a reduction in red blood cells. Vitamin B12 is normally produced in the horses gut.
Fish meals are used in compound feeds to supplement B12.
Alfalfa.

Folic Acid
Folic acid is linked to vitamin B12 and is vital in the production of red blood cells. A deficiency can cause anaemia and poor growth. A supplement of vitamin B12 can help in cases of a folic acid deficiency. Good quality grass, hay and oil seeds contain folic acid.

Biotin
Biotin is a vitamin containing sulphur. It is involved in protein, fat and carbohydrate metabolism. A lack of biotin can lead to poor skin and hoof growth. It is commonly supplemented for the horse with poor feet where it can help in strengthening the hoof and promoting growth.
Bladderwrack, Coltsfoot, Eyebright, Fennel, Garlic, Marigold, Meadowsweet, Nettles, Red Clover, Rosehips.

Choline
An essential vitamin for helping to build and maintain cell structure. Deficiency reduces growth rate and can effect liver function. Choline is distributed extensively in feedstuff and is high in green forage and yeast.
Aniseed, Comfrey, Dandelion, Nettles, Parsley, Raspberry.

Fat Soluble Vitamins

Vitamin A (Retinol)
Carotene, which is the pigment found in carrots and other plants, is rich in vitamin A. This is necessary for vision, growth, resistance to disease and reproduction. It also helps maintain healthy mucus membranes. A deficiency can cause eye damage, poor growth and reproductive failure. Green leafy forages as well as carrots are rich in Vitamin A.
Alfalfa, Bladderwrack, Comfrey, Couch Grass, Dandelion, Fennel, Fenugreek, Garlic, Marigold, Marshmallow, Mint, Nettles, Parsley, Rosehips.

Vitamin C (Ascorbic Acid)
Vitamin C helps in the formation and maintenance of collagen which is vital to the structure of skin and connective tissue. A deficiency can slow down healing and cause weight loss. Green leafy forages contain high levels of vitamin C as do citrus fruits.
Alfalfa, Bladderwrack, Coltsfoot, Dandelion, Fenugreek, Garlic, Hawthorn, Meadowsweet, Nettles, Oregano, Parsley, Raspberry, Rosehips, Seaweed, Strawberry, Wormwood.

Vitamin D (Calciferol)
Vitamin D helps the body in the absorption of calcium and phosphorus. Deficiency or excess amounts of vitamin D can cause swollen joints, lameness and impaired growth. Vitamin D occurs as two pro vitamins converted to the vitamin through the sunlight on the skin. This vitamin is not common in plants. Colostrum is a rich source of vitamin D to the newly born foal.
Oil containing seeds and *Alfalfa, Bladderwrack, Dandelion.*

Vitamin E (Tocopherol)
Vitamin E is an anti-oxidant. It acts with selenium in maintaining the stability of red blood cells and the vascular system. A deficiency can cause problems to the heart and skeletal system as well as affecting fertility. Poor quality feed and stress will increase the vitamin E requirement.
Most green fodder and some cereal grains, as well as the following herbs, are rich in vitamin E:
Alfalfa, Bladderwrack, Dandelion, Fenugreek, Red Clover.

Vitamin K
Vitamin K is essential for blood clotting and a deficiency will increase the time it takes for blood to clot.
Alfalfa, Rosehips and Green leafy plants.

OTHER HERBAL PREPARATIONS

INFUSION

This method is sometimes helpful where a horse is a poor eater and it is necessary to ensure that herbs are fed.

An infusion is a beverage made like tea, by combining boiling water with the plants (usually the green parts or the flowers) to extract their active ingredients. The boiling water is poured over the plants or they can be added to boiling water after it has been removed from the heat. For feeding in liquid form, strain the infusion into a cup. If necessary sugar or honey can be added to improve the taste. Normally you should use the infusion warm or cool but to induce sweating or to break up a cough use it as hot as can be taken without causing it to burn the mouth. Herb teas can be taken over a period of time in small regular doses. The daily dose usually ranges from 2 to 4 cups, depending on the severity of the problem, the potency of the plant and the size of the horse. Use 15-20 gms of herb to a cup of water

Where the liquid is being added to the normal feed it is not necessary to strain it unless the horse will not eat it. If the horse will not eat it the strained liquid can be syringed into the mouth.

DECOCTION

Although this method is time consuming the resulting liquid usually gives a quicker response because it will extract primarily the mineral salts and bitter principles of plants, rather than vitamins and volatile ingredients. Roots, bark and seeds require boiling to extract their active ingredients. Boil about 20 gms (0.7 oz) plant parts per cup of water. Green plant parts can be added to cold water and boiled for 3 to 4 minutes or they can be added to boiling water and boiled for the same time. You should cover the pot whilst it is boiling. Hard materials need boiling for about 10 minutes to extract their properties. Strain out the plant parts before using the decoction although the remaining herb parts can also be used in the horses feed. Use 2 to 3 cups daily.

TINCTURE
Add approximately 120 gm (4oz) of powdered herb, depending on the plant's potency, to 500ml. (1 pint) of alcohol. Add water to make a 50% alcohol solution, stand for two or three weeks, shaking daily, then strain and pour the liquid into a bottle suitable for storage. Tinctures will keep for a long time due to the alcohol content. Homeopaths use very dilute tinctures as their basic medicinal preparations.

POWDER
You can grind dried plant parts into powder by hand or by using a blender. Powder can be taken with water, milk or sprinkled on food.

ESSENCE
Dissolve one ounce of the herb's essential oil in a pint of alcohol. This will preserve the volatile essential oils of many plants, which are generally not soluble in water.

OINTMENT
Mix one part of the remedy in powdered form with four parts of hot petroleum jelly or a similar substance. An old method is to boil the ingredients in water until the desired properties are extracted (as decoction). Strain the liquid, add the liquid to vegetable oil, and simmer until the water has completely evaporated. Beeswax can be added to achieve a firm consistency. Heat the mixture slowly, and stir until completely blended.

POULTICE
A poultice is used to apply a remedy externally to a skin area with moist heat. To prepare, crush the medicinal parts of the plant to a pulp and heat. Moisten the materials by mixing with a hot substance such as bread and milk. Apply directly to the skin. A good way is to spread the paste or pulp on a wet, hot cloth, apply, and wrap the cloth around to help retain moisture and heat. Where irritant plants are involved keep the paste between two pieces of cloth to prevent direct contact with the skin; after removing the poultice, wash the area well with water or herb tea to remove any residue.

AROMATHERAPY

The term Aromatherapy was first used by French chemist Rene Maurice Gattefosse in 1928 to describe the therapeutic use of essences and oils extracted from plants. In fact the qualities and benefits of plant extracts date back over 5000 years when they were in common use by the early Egyptians. It is the same principle of essential oils extracted from plants that are used in Aromatherapy today.

There are various means of treatment using Aromatherapy including adding essential oils to bath water, inhalation or, more commonly in the case of horses, by gently massaging the oils into the skin. This encourages the absorbtion of the oils into the body tissue where they are dispersed to treat local infections, as well as stimulating the body's own defences.

Essential oils have antibacterial antiviral and anti-inflammatory properties. These were widely used to prevent and fight infection during both world wars.

The method of extracting essential oils depends on where in the plant the oil is situated. In most cases distillation is used. With this method fresh or dried flowers are packed tight in a still and steam is passed through it. During this process the oil evaporates into steam and when cooled the essential oils will separate from the water.

Some plants can simply be squeezed to extract the essential oils and this can be done either by hand or by using a press.

Other processes can involve soaking in hot oil or other liquids but the object remains the same in all cases, to extract the highest quality essential oils from the plants in question. These oils are then diluted before use. Essential oils should not be taken orally unless specifically prescribed to do so. Externally they can be extremely effective for a number of conditions particularly relating to the skin.

Many essential oils are very strong substances and they can be dangerous if incorrectly used. Some will affect sensitive skin whilst others should not be used for pregnant mares. For this reason you should always obtain the advice of a qualified aromatherapist and veterinary surgeon before undertaking treatment using aromatherapy.

HOMEOPATHY

The name Homeopathy is derived from the Greek words Homoios meaning 'like' and Pathos meaning 'suffering' but the man credited with its discovery is German scientist Samuel Christian Hahnemann who studied medicine in the late 18th century.

Hahnemann found that by taking repeated doses of quinine into his otherwise healthy body he produced symptoms of malaria, the very same disease that quinine was used to treat. Once he stopped taking the quinine the symptoms went and he returned to good health. This experiment convinced Hahnemann as to the basic principal of Homeopathy that "like can be cured by like".

Further research satisfied Hahnemann as to the validity of his findings but he was concerned that some of the remedies that he had developed were toxic. In an effort to reduce toxic levels Hahnemann experimented by diluting his remedies. It is this aspect that is most surprising and that many people began to doubt about his theory. For Hahnemann found that the medical power of his remedy increased in proportion to its dilution.

The method used to prepare a remedy to this theory is for one part of a substance to be diluted with nine parts of a neutral substance such as water or pure alcohol (decimal) or with ninety nine parts (centesimal). This is shaken in a precise method and the resulting mixture is called the first potency. When one part of this potency is diluted further by nine, or ninety nine parts the result is called the second potency and so on. This process can continue so that the resulting dilution (potency) only contains the original material at a sub molecular level.

Such dilution means that many substances can be used that would normally be too toxic and the theory that Hahnemann had discovered was that there remained an influence from the original substances that has the potential to effect the physiology of the body.

BACH FLOWER REMEDIES

These are named after Dr Edward Bach the physician who developed this form of therapy. Whilst practicing orthodox medicine Dr Bach began to question the practice of treating only the symptoms of the disease and looked for a way to treat the mind and body as a whole. He spent some time researching homeopathy and developed a number of medicines based on those principles.

Bach discovered that there was a relationship between the state of mind of the patient and the treatment required. He believed that it was possible to restore harmony to the mind and the body, which would encourage a state of self healing. In keeping with his interest in homeopathy Bach looked to plant extracts to develop his range of 38 flower remedies which he related to seven emotional states. A 39th remedy comprises of a blend of five from the 38 (Cherry Plum, Clematis, Impatiens, Rock Rose and Star of Bethlehem) to become Rescue Remedy, the most well known of Bach flower remedies. Only a few drops are required and these can be added to a treat or water.

These remedies are safe to use for both horse and rider and will not interfere with conventional medicine.

Many people find Bach flower remedies of great benefit particularly for shock, anxiety or stress.

McTIMONEY CHIROPRACTIC

McTimoney Chiropractic is a unique branch of the chiropractic profession in the UK. The technique is named after its originator John McTimoney, who developed his whole-body style of treatment from those techniques originally taught at the first college of chiropractic, the Palmer College, founded in the closing years of the last century by D.D. Palmer, the originator of chiropractic.

Like people, animals suffer from back, neck, pelvic and musculo-skeletal problems, and, like us, they can benefit from McTimoney Chiropractic manipulation.

For over 40 years McTimoney Animal Chiropractors have been helping a variety of animals, especially horses and dogs with a non-invasive technique of manipulation that aligns and balances the whole body, with special attention being paid to the spine and pelvis. It helps to both restore and maintain health, soundness and performance. It works holistically to eliminate the cause, not just to treat the symptoms.

The treatment itself consists of a qualified practitioner analysing the animal's spine, pelvis and other relevant joints for any misalignments or spasm in the associated muscles. The problem areas are treated with precise and rapid adjustments to correct the misalignment and reduce muscle spasm. Practitioners use only their hands for analysis and adjustment.

The aftercare of the animal often includes rest and/or limited exercise for a few days and depending on the severity of the problem several treatments may be required, with yearly or twice yearly check-ups advised both to help achieve optimum performance and as a preventative measure.

Practitioners rely on owners observations and referrals from veterinary surgeons as to when an animal requires treatment. Indications often include: -

- Lameness after a fall or other accident where alternative causes have been ruled out.
- Uncharacteristic changes in performance, behaviour or temperament.
- Limb-dragging or odd/irregular action.
- Absence of any resolution of the problem, using conventional methods.
- Unlevelness especially behind.
- Uneven wear of shoes.
- Sore or 'cold' backs: uneven pressure from saddles, numnahs etc.
- Uneven muscle development or atrophy.
- Asymmetry, such as stiffness on one rein, or a disunited canter.
- Recurrence of symptoms previously successfully treated by chiropractic manipulation.

The most obvious cause for many of the above symptoms is trauma, for example falls, accidents, slips and getting cast. But even subtle causes can also be to blame, for example, conformation problems, e.g. long or weak backs, ill-fitting equipment, excess weight and even dental and shoeing problems.

It is very important that before a McTimoney Chiropractic treatment is given the owner has consulted his/her veterinary surgeon, as it is illegal for a non-veterinary chiropractic practitioner to treat your animal without veterinary approval. At just over 50 years old McTimoney Chiropractic is a relative newcomer to the world of chiropractic, offering a refined, effective and safe treatment developed from mainstream chiropractic based on sound chiropractic principles.

SECTION FOUR

The Digestive System	137
The Respiratory System	153
The Circulatory System	161
The Urinary System	167
The Coat and Skin	169
The Muscular and Skeletal System	181
The Reproductive System	193
Behaviour	203
Box Rest	211
Eyes	212

THE DIGESTIVE SYSTEM

A Brief Description	138
Appetite	139
Colic	140
Spasmodic Colic	140
Impactive Colic	141
Gaseous Colic	141
Sand Colic	142
Twisted Gut	142
Constipation	143
Grass Sickness	143
Diarrhoea	144
Weight Loss	145
Dehydration	145
Sweating	146
The Liver	146
Worms	147
Threadworms	147
Roundworms	148
Redworm	148
Pinworms	149
Lungworm	149
Tapeworm	150
Bots	150
Management & Treatment	150

A BRIEF DESCRIPTION OF THE DIGESTIVE SYSTEM

A horse is a herbivore, which means he will naturally eat herbs and vegetables, and his digestive system is designed to allow this. An adult horse has 40 or 42 teeth, which enable him to grasp and grind vegetation into a digestible pulp. The food is pushed backwards with the tongue into the gullet. The soft palate blocks off the nose and the larynx closes, so that the food cannot leak into the respiratory tract. Food material enters the stomach through a one-way muscular valve, which prevents the horse from regurgitating. This is the reason why it is said that a horse cannot be sick. When the food is in the stomach enzymes and acids are produced to help with the digestion. It then passes through a valve into the small intestine; a long muscular tube known as the gut. As the food passes through, the small intestine fluids produced by the liver, pancreas and intestinal glands help to break it down into fats, proteins and carbohydrates. These are absorbed into the bloodstream and transported to the body to produce energy and various materials required for development.

As the food passes on into the large colon the natural bacteria helps to break down the cellulose into its basic constituents. It is here that a considerable amount of water is absorbed, and as the digested food continues through the small colon the process of electrolyte and water absorption continues. The progression is then to the rectum where the waste material (dung) passes through to the outside environment.

APPETITE

It is often a sign that all is not well when a horse loses its appetite and there can be a number of reasons. If the loss of appetite is due to disease or infection there are usually other signs. Horses, like people will often go off their food when they are ill and a veterinary examination will establish the cause.

Loss of appetite can also be due to a change of climate, management or exercise. Competition horses may still be "wound up" and unenthusiastic about eating after returning from the sport. Once it is established that there are no clinical reasons for loss of appetite there are ways of encouraging a horse to eat.

A horse needs to be relaxed and as free of stress as possible. Sometimes the mental change of allowing a horse to pick at some good grass is helpful, even where this has to be carried out in controlled circumstances with the horse "in hand".

Sometimes after racing or strenuous exercise it may be necessary to relax the horses digestive system before it will begin to eat. This can be achieved by making an **infusion** of **carminative** herbs such as **Chamomile.** It can be easier to get a horse to take liquid until the appetite is restored. Usually within hours a horse will begin to relax and start to eat. At this stage other dried herbs can be added to a small amount of food. These can include **Chamomile, Valerian** and **Hops**. As the appetite improves the food can be gradually increased. It is important that the quantity of food is gradually increased to normal rations. Some horses are picky, fussy types and are never very enthusiastic about eating. In such cases it is important to find the most appetising feed that will suit the particular requirements of that horse. Most good feed companies have nutritionists to help and advise and they will usually provide samples.

There are also herbs to improve the appeal of food and help stimulate appetite. Mixing **Mint** or **Fenugreek** with feed is often successful, also grated carrot or apple can be used.

Authors Note:
It has always been our policy to remove feed after a reasonable time if a horse does not eat it, maybe after 2 to 3 hours. Leaving old food in the manger does not make it more appetising. Also if a meal is left for a horse to just pick at continually it makes it less likely that there will be any more enthusiasm when the next meal arrives. Better to feed little and often, but to clear the manger after each meal. There is nothing nicer than to be greeted by an enthusiastic horse at feed time.

COLIC

Colic is a term used to describe **abdominal pain**.

The degree of colic and the number of causes can vary greatly and in all cases it is important to consult a veterinary surgeon since colic can be a most serious problem.

Many forms of colic are avoidable with good management. For example colic can be bought about by lack of exercise, feeding too quickly after exercise, a lack of sufficient water, poor diet, internal damage resulting from a poor **worming** programme, eating excessive amounts of straw bedding and various similar preventable causes.

SPASMODIC COLIC

The most common form of colic is spasmodic colic, the symptoms of this are usually a moderately distressed horse showing signs of sweating, constantly lying down and getting up, maybe looking at its flanks and kicking at its abdomen. In some cases horses will roll and there is a danger of them becoming **cast**. Usually there are few droppings with spasmodic colic but the condition can come and go very quickly. The cause of spasmodic colic is not always easy to identify, although it is widely believed that the most likely reason for unidentified recurring spasmodic colic is caused by **Redworm**. The normal treatment that a veterinary surgeon would apply for spasmodic colic is to administer a **relaxant** or **spasmolytic** drug. There are herbs that will help prevent spasmodic colic, but they should be fed as a preventative rather than a treatment since **the incidence of colic should be dealt with as a matter of urgency and a veterinary surgeon should be consulted**. Whatever herbs are fed they will not replace good management.

There are **anthelmintic** herbs that will help prevent worm damage the most common being **Garlic**. This can be extremely good in helping to prevent worms and can be fed on a regular basis as a supplement to the diet.

IMPACTIVE COLIC

Impactive colic is where an impaction of food material causes an obstruction in the large intestine. This can be caused by the horse eating an excessive amount of straw bedding or having free access to large amounts of food. A horse may demonstrate less pain with an impactive colic than with **spasmodic colic**. Typically the horse may tend to lie down and look off colour without the signs of any violent pain, often getting up and down and looking at its flanks.

A veterinary surgeon can normally examine and locate the cause of any obstruction. Often in the case of an impaction a vet will "tube" a horse to administer large volumes of liquid paraffin with salt water through a stomach tube. A veterinary surgeon may apply an **analgesic** drug to help ease discomfort as nature takes it course in clearing the impaction.

GASEOUS COLIC

A more unusual colic can be the result of a build up of gas in the intestines. There can be several causes for this and it is usually very painful. The horse will show signs of severe abdominal pain, sweating and often violent rolling. The build up of gas may occur in front of an impaction or can be due to a major obstruction such as where the intestine has become twisted (**twisted gut**). Gas distension of the stomach and intestine can occur if food material ferments within the intestine, for example, when grass cuttings are used as a feed. Relief is sometimes achieved by the veterinary surgeon inserting a tube into the stomach to allow gases to escape.

SAND COLIC
This is a problem that is more likely to occur in a sandy or dusty climate where there can be a gradual build up of sand passing through the digestive system which collects in the large intestine and can lead to **impactive colic**. In some cases the weight of the sand can result in a **twisted gut**. Usually the sand is taken in when a horse is on poor grazing, on sandy surfaces or is eating off of the floor. The build up may take some time whilst the weight of the sand prevents food passing through the system and allows it to accumulate in a vulnerable position. Where there is a risk of sand colic there are herbs that can help in its prevention if added to the daily diet. **Psyllium** is best known for this which together with **Marshmallow** can help the sand in its passage through the system. However, it must be stressed that these are a dietary aid in preventing sand colic and not a cure once it occurs.
As in all cases of colic a veterinary surgeon should attend.

TWISTED GUT
Probably the most serious and dramatic colic is that of a twisted gut, which in simple terms is where a piece of intestine is twisted or folded to cause obstruction of the blood supply. The horse usually shows signs of severe pain and sweating and can often be violent and uncontrollable because of the severity of the pain. **This is a very serious condition and early expert veterinary help is required.** It is not normal for this condition to correct itself although in some cases a skilful veterinary surgeon may be able to help. As a last resort, the veterinary surgeon may be able to carry out abdominal surgery. This often represents the best chance of survival for a horse with this condition. Even when surgery is carried out it is sometimes not possible to save the horse.

CONSTIPATION

Constipation in horses should be avoided. The first rule is that a good clean fresh water supply should always be available to the horse. Also by paying attention to any changes in dung, it is usually possible to adjust the diet to prevent problems before they become serious. Constipation can be an indication of **impactive colic** which requires immediate veterinary attention.

In some cases constipation leading to **colic** type symptoms can be an indication of **grass sickness.** Where there is a change in the droppings and they become firmer this is an indication that some action is required. By adjusting the diet it is often possible to prevent these changes which can lead to constipation or even **colic**. Some herbs that include **laxative** qualities are **Dandelion, Fenugreek** and **Valerian.** These can be fed individually or a combination of them will offer an excellent blend that can be added to the daily feed.

The practice of adding sunflower or other natural oils to the feed occasionally can also help in the prevention of constipation.

GRASS SICKNESS

As the name suggests this is a disease that affects horses or ponies at grass and although the cause is still unknown the symptoms of grass sickness are similar to **constipation** and **colic.** Horses suffering from this may also have trembling of the muscles in the shoulder, quarters or neck, other signs can include rapid loss of coordination. Grass Sickness is a little understood disease and often by the time it is diagnosed it has become life threatening. However, there have been cases where veterinary treatment has been successful. A case that comes to mind is the winner of the 2,000 guineas Mr. Baileys. After suffering this life threatening disease he went on to a successful stud career in Kentucky. This is a good example where early attention saved the life of the horse. There has been some very good research carried out on grass sickness and this is ongoing. Since the greatest incidence of this disease is in Scotland it is not surprising that the Equine Grass Sickness Fund is based there. This organisation can provide further information.

DIARRHOEA

Diarrhoea is often the result of **inflammation** of the intestines, which is known as **enteritis**. This can be caused through nutrition, **parasitic infestation** or other internal infections.

Where the diarrhoea appears to be through nutritional causes probably the best action is to just feed good hay and clean water for a few days. If the diarrhoea continues for more than twenty four hours it is worth having an investigation carried out by your veterinary surgeon.

Where it is necessary to investigate for parasitic problems, a dropping sample can be taken and sent away for analysis. This can also be checked for bacteria and it can be helpful in forming an overall opinion as to the state of the horse's **digestive system**.

If the problem is through parasitic invasion then **anthelmintic** herbs can be helpful. Most vets will advise on a **worming** programme. Bacterial problems are more difficult to deal with and a veterinary surgeon may prescribe **antibiotics**. In all cases of diarrhoea it is important to ensure that sufficient fluid intake is maintained and in some cases a vet may choose to do this **intravenously**.

There are a number of cases where diarrhoea appears to have no specific cause. Although some can be treated with drugs often these are not effective. We have experienced, on a number of occasions, horses that have developed diarrhoea after undertaking a course of **antibiotics**. This has had an adverse affect on their **digestive system** and through that their **immune system**. We have successfully dealt with a number of horses in this condition by feeding **Raspberry**. These have had the affect of increasing the bacteria in the gut that may have been destroyed by the **antibiotics**. Often within two or three days of feeding **Raspberry** a great improvement is found.
(See also **foal scour**.)

WEIGHT LOSS

Various problems with the digestive system, as well as a number of serious diseases, can result in weight loss and **it is important to identify the cause**. The inability to absorb nutrients from the feed can result in weight loss and this can be due to the presence of **parasites** or as a result of severe previous **parasite damage**. Persistent **diarrhoea** will also result in weight loss. Once the cause, or the disease that is responsible for the condition has been identified, there is a good chance that herbs can play a useful part.

DEHYDRATION

Dehydration is caused by an insufficient water supply to maintain correct body fluid function. This can result from insufficient intake of water or through excessive losses such as in the case of **sweating** or **diarrhoea**.

Also certain ailments and diseases can impair correct fluid balance such as **kidney** malfunction. In many cases dehydration is the result of insufficient water intake whilst undertaking excessive exercise or through extreme heat, thus resulting in heavy **sweating**. Great losses of fluids upset the delicate balance of body salts including **magnesium**, **sodium**, **potassium** and **calcium**. In such cases **electrolytes** should be fed to both promote the intake of water and help restore the lost body salts.

A good clean water supply is fundamental to a horse's well being and it is important to take note of the normal drinking habits of each horse to ensure that any changes are noted at an early stage.

An easy test for dehydration is to pinch the skin on a horses neck using a thumb and forefinger. This should have some elasticity to it and when released will spring back into place. If it is slow to do so it could indicate dehydration.

Electrolytes can be fed according to need through a training programme, particularly after a race or strenuous exercise.

Herbs can be very useful in the balance of body fluids and salts and one of the best known common herbs is **Dandelion**. Although usually regarded as a diuretic **Dandelion** is unique in that it is very high in **potassium** and **magnesium** and it will help replace these naturally.

SWEATING

Sweating is a part of the body's cooling system and a normal function of a healthy horse, although excessive sweating can result in loss of body salts and **dehydration**.

Sweating for no apparent reason can be a response to pain, discomfort or **anxiousness** and the cause should be investigated. Sometimes a horse may appear not to sweat even after strenuous exercise and the use of a **diophoretic** herb can help induce sweat. The best known herb with this characteristic is **Garlic** and it can routinely be added to the daily feed as a good all round herb.

THE LIVER

The liver is the largest **gland** in the body. It weighs about 5 kgs (11 lbs) in an adult horse. About three quarters of the **blood** passing through the liver comes through a vein from the intestines and contains remnants of digested food that have been absorbed through the wall of the gut. The remaining **blood** passes into the liver, through a main artery, to provide nourishment to the liver cells.

Blood is effectively "filtered" through the liver and it passes to the heart. The liver has a duct, which carries **bile** into the duodenum because the horse has no gall bladder. In the natural state a horse eats continuously and passes **bile** continuously and has no reason to store it.

The liver cleanses the **blood** of noxious substances, such as drugs and poisons and excretes **bile** into the intestine. It helps govern the metabolic process and in regulating **blood** levels of **carbohydrates**, **protein** and **fat** and the storage of sugar and **vitamins**, which it helps to deliver into the bloodstream.

The livers ability to transform and convert various substances can help protect the body against poisons by changing them into harmless ones that the body can deal with.

Most conditions of the liver result from infections through other parts of the body such as the **digestive system**. Symptoms of liver disease include **jaundice**, **weight loss** and **diarrhoea**. There can also be swelling resulting from a build up of fluid in the abdomen, chest and legs. See **glandular system**.

Liver damage can result from contamination of **roundworm** larvae as it passes through the digestive process.

Cholagogue and **Hepatic** herbs can have a positive effect on the liver. Among the herbs that are considered to make a good liver tonic are; **Milk Thistle, Burdock** and **Dandelion**.

WORMS

Worm control is a vital part of horse management since neglect can result in serious internal damage that can have a long term and life threatening effect.

It is not always apparent when horses have become affected by worms and by the time that there are noticeable signs there probably already is some internal damage.

Different types of worms can affect horses at different stages of their life and it is important to have some understanding of these factors.

THREADWORMS
(Ascarrids, Strongyloides western)
Threadworms are often passed to a foal through the mares milk. The adult worms live in the small intestine and infection can cause **scouring** in foals – usually coinciding with the time that the mare has her **foaling heat**. A good worming programme in the mare can help and the foal itself can be treated for threadworm when it is at least a week old.

ROUNDWORMS
(Parascaris equorum)
This is another worm that can invade the foal up to the age of 2 years when it develops a resistance to this parasite. The infective larvae is eaten by the foal and then hatches in the foals gut. An adult female can lay up to 1 million eggs a day in the small intestine of the young horse and when they hatch they migrate through the bloodstream to the **liver** and lungs. This causes the foal to cough up the larvae. When they are then swallowed they develop into adults and begin the egg laying cycle inside the intestine. It takes 2 to 3 months from when a foal eats the eggs until the larvae matures and eggs are passed out in the foals droppings into the stable or field.

It takes about a month for these eggs to develop into infective larvae starting the whole process again. These worms can grow as long as 30 cm (12") and anything up to 1000 can accumulate in the foals gut.

Visible signs of contamination are **weight loss**, poor coat and a pot-belly appearance. Invasion causes slow growth through infection and in severe cases can block the small intestine completely resulting in serious damage or death.

Good paddock management is crucial and even more important with mares and foals since the invasion of roundworms often begins in contaminated paddocks. Ideally paddocks should be kept clean and rotated so that they are rested for a year at a time.

REDWORMS
Large strongyles (Strongylus vulgaris) and **Small strongyles** (Trichonema species).
Both of these groups have a similar life cycle. The adult worm lays eggs in the large intestine of the horse which are passed out in the droppings. Large strongyles are coloured red from the blood that they suck. They can be up to 8 cms (3") long. Small strongyles are white and are up to 2.5 cms (1") long. Eggs can stay on a paddock for up to a year where the larvae develops and can be eaten by the horse whilst it is grazing. It then passes into the intestine where the small strongyles will burrow into

the large intestine and either remain dormant, or emerge 2 or 3 months later as egg laying adults. Several generations of larvae can be passed through into the paddock in one season causing high levels of contamination. The strongylus vulgaris larvae migrates throughout the body through artery walls where it can cause damage and blockage that may interrupt the blood supply to the gut resulting in **colic**.

It is believed that Redworm may be the most likely cause in many cases of recurring **spasmodic colic**. The mature larvae eventually return into the gut and become egg laying adults 5 to 9 months after original infection.

The larvae of **strongylus edentatus** migration takes them through the large intestine and the **liver** to the lining of the abdomen returning to the large intestine to become egg laying adults 5-12 months after entering the horse. These worms feed off the gut wall and cause **ulcers** and irritation. Redworms can affect all ages.

PINWORMS
(Oxyuris equi, seatworm)
Adults can grow up to 10 cms (4"). They live in the large intestine. The female lays her eggs near the anus which often causes irritation and itching. The larvae develop within 4 days and the eggs fall onto the pasture where they are eaten by the grazing horse. The larvae develop in the large intestine wall for up to 5 months before becoming egg laying adults. Pinworms are not normally a serious problem because routine wormers usually kill them.

LUNGWORMS
(Dictyocaulus arnfieldi)
It would seem that lungworm is not common in horses and even badly affected horses do not pass eggs or larvae in their droppings, making it difficult to diagnose. As the name suggest lungworm can affect the air passages and cause a **chronic** cough, particularly during exercise.

About 70% of donkeys have lungworm and horses can become infected when grazing with them.

TAPEWORMS
(Anoplocephala perfoliata)
The adult greyish-white worm is up to 8 cms (3") long. It lives in the lower part of the small intestine and in the large intestine of the horse. The adult tapeworm continuously grow segments containing eggs that are passed out to the pasture in the droppings. The eggs are eaten by oribatid mites that live in the grass and the tapeworm develops as a microscopic cyst in the body of the mites. The horse becomes infected through eating the mite whilst grazing. Large numbers of tapeworms may cause **diarrhoea** and damage to the small intestine.

BOTS
The bot fly lays its yellowish eggs on the hairs of the horse during summer months, normally on the legs, shoulders and neck areas. The bots are ingested by the horse licking itself and they hatch into a maggot like larvae as they pass to the stomach and mature. They pass out in droppings the following spring 8-10 months later. The larvae take between 3 and 5 weeks to hatch as adult flys hence completing the cycle.

MANAGEMENT AND TREATMENT
Worms are an unwelcome parasite in the horse and we should do all we can to reduce the incidence of invasion. Herbs can be extremely helpful as part of an overall management programme and there are many people who successfully control worms using completely natural methods and substances. Such a programme requires extreme care in every aspect of horse management and diet, which in most cases is not achievable. Because of the importance of good worm control, we would rather use correctly prepared proprietary products than compromise the horses well being. However, even when using standard **wormers** there is still much that can be done to minimise the incidence of worms.

Much is said on the need to have good clean grazing. This cannot be overstated. Most worm infections start from eggs being ingested by the grazing horse. If it were possible to remove all of these from the paddocks the problem would almost cease. A good start therefore is to remove all droppings every day. In most cases the eggs are sitting in them. Of course it is idealistic to say do not overgraze and rest fields for a year between grazing. As our horse numbers increase the available grazing reduces in both quantity and quality. However there are methods of natural management that can greatly help. For example rotation of grazing areas for different animals can reduce contamination. Sheep and cattle have been used for this purpose by knowledgeable farmers over many years. Good grassland management is also important, such as harrowing, topping and even reseeding.

An important part of the programme is to ensure that all horses are treated for worms before they are turned out. This will reduce the contamination in the field. Also all horses sharing grazing should be wormed at the same time – usually every 4 – 6 weeks.

Anthelmintic herbs can be helpful – however, some of them are now on the poison list and should not be used by the layman. Thankfully there are some that can be used safely, the best known of which is **Garlic.** Add every day in the horses feed and it not only helps in the prevention of worms but it will also help to repel insects such as bots from depositing their eggs on the horse.

THE RESPIRATORY SYSTEM

The Respiratory System	154
Nasal Discharge	155
Sinus Discharge	155
Nasal Food Discharges	156
Nasal Haemorrhaging	156
Viral Infections	157
Bacterial Infections	157
C.O.P.D.	158
Pneumonia	159
Pleurisy	160

THE RESPIRATORY SYSTEM

The normal respiratory rate of a horse is ten to fourteen breaths per minute. Various factors affect the respiratory rate such as exercise, excitement, environment and of course disease.

Breathing air into the lungs provides oxygen through the bloodstream to the muscles and organs of the body. The respiratory system also expels the carbon dioxide as a waste product, thus maintaining a cycle of providing new oxygen throughout the body. Air enters the nostrils and passes through the nasal passages to what is known as the upper respiratory tract.

This system allows the passage of large volumes of air to pass to the lungs using an ingenious path of biological valves and compartments that adjust to open and close the pathway for food into the digestive system as the requirements for intake of air increases.

At the back of the mouth the soft palate is relaxed allowing the passage of air whilst the larynx acts as a valve in reducing the channel for food into the digestive system. This allows the maximum flow of air into connected cavities known as the sinuses which are filled with air as it passes on through the trachea (windpipe).

This unique system adjusts to the passage of air as the requirements increase during exercise. Any ailment or disease that causes the blocking or reduction of airways will obviously reduce airflow and have an effect on the well being and performance of the competition horse.

The most obvious sign of infection is a **nasal discharge**, usually **mucus**. In some cases this may show **pus**, **blood** or even food and it is important to establish the nature and cause of any discharge so that correct veterinary treatment can be carried out.

NASAL DISCHARGE

It is normal for a horse to produce a small amount of **mucus** and this can discharge from both nostrils usually after exercise. Abnormal discharges of **mucus** or **pus** are usually associated with a cough **(C.O.P.D.)**.

SINUS DISCHARGE

These are often from one nostril and can be a foul smelling **pus** as a result of a dental or other infection. This can cause blockage and swelling of the area thus reducing airflow.

Occasionally a discharge can be due to a **cyst** or more unusually a **tumour** which can obstruct a nasal passage. Where a discharge is apparent from both nostrils, it results from further back in the respiratory tract such as an infection of the **guttural pouch**. This may be a **fungal infection** which often causes severe nosebleeds as well as a foul smelling discharge. This can be a serious disease and like all respiratory discharges should be investigated by a veterinary surgeon to establish the cause.

Investigation is now made easier with the use of fibre optic endoscopic examination equipment. This allows for the internal examination of the respiratory tract by the vet. Commonly known as the **endoscope** this instrument helps to achieve an accurate diagnosis of most diseases that affect the respiratory system.

When a discharge is related to **fungal infection** the best herbs to feed are **Thyme**, **Red Clover** and **Golden Rod** all of which have **antifungal** qualities. As with all disorders of the respiratory system, **Garlic** should be included in the blend and **Echinacea** is excellent to help build up the **immune system** to fight the infection. Where a **tumour** is causing obstruction to the nasal passage, it may require surgical removal to quickly re-establish sufficient airways. The same herbs have proven helpful for **tumours** but they do take time to get into the system.

Very occasionally a **nasal discharge** can be caused by an infection resulting from some foreign body getting stuck in the nasal canal. A twig or similar item can become lodged and in some cases require surgical removal.

NASAL FOOD DISCHARGE

The most common cause of nasal discharge of food is **choke** or an obstruction of the **digestive system**. Other obstructions in the throat can cause a difficulty in breathing, and may cause a discharge of food or water through the nostrils. The obstruction may be due to an **abscess** (**strangles**) or **tumour**.

Where milk runs from the nostrils of a young foal it can be due to a defect in the respiratory or digestive system. It is important to establish the cause early since the likelihood of **pneumonia** in such cases is high.

NASAL HAEMORRHAGING (EPISTAXIS)

The most common cause of bleeding from nostrils (usually both) in a horse is Exercise Induced Pulmonary Haemorrhage (**E.I.P.H.**) commonly known as **bursting** or **bleeding**. It is usually the result of strenuous exercise or racing.

Forceful breathing during exercise causes stress to the lungs resulting in damage to the tissue and haemorrhaging. The incidence of this condition is probably greater than most people realise. Post race endoscopic examinations have shown a number of horses **burst** or **bleed** without the manifestation of **blood** discharging.

The presence of an inherent respiratory condition increases the likelihood of **bleeding** which can affect any breed of horse.

The resulting damage to the lungs can take as little as ten days to several months to improve and repair, depending on the severity of the damage, subsequent treatment and management.

When using herbs to help with **E.I.P.H.** you should feed those that help alleviate any underlying respiratory disorders (see **C.O.P.D.**) as well as those that will help to repair and restore the tissues and capillaries of the lungs. These may include **Horsetail**, **Marigold**, **Fenugreek**, **Slippery Elm**, **Marshmallow** and **Comfrey**.

VIRAL INFECTIONS
Equine Influenza
Viruses will spread rapidly in horses, through stabling, transporting and other close contact. The most common viral infections affecting horses are Equine Influenza and **Equine Hepevirus**. Most horses are vaccinated against Equine Influenza. The symptoms are high temperature and coughing with a watery nasal discharge. It usually takes 2 to 3 weeks to recover from Equine Influenza.

Equine Hepevirus is a respiratory infection, which is commonly regarded as a **stable cough**. Other strains of this virus (**E.H.V.I. subtype 1**) can cause mares to abort (**Rhinopneumonitis**). Although not common, this is an extremely serious condition that is contagious and must be reported. Most mares are now vaccinated against **Rhinopneumonitis**. Symptoms include an intermittent cough and a snotty nose, loss of **appetite** and high temperature. In older horses a **nasal discharge** may be the only sign of infection.

Where viral infections affect the respiratory system, herbs that will help expel **mucus** and relax the airways can be fed. **Garlic**, **Liquorice**, **Thyme** and **Red clover** should be included and **Echinacea**, **Mint** and **St Johns Wort** can all be considered for their **antiviral** qualities.

BACTERIAL INFECTIONS
Bacteria normally enters the body through inhalation or open wounds. It is common for bacteria to be present in the respiratory tract and it normally only becomes a problem when other factors such as stress or a **virus** are present. In some instances bacterial infections can be the primary cause of infection such as **strangles**. Severe infections invariably involve the lungs and result in **pneumonia**.

As with all respiratory infections, **Red Clover**, **Garlic**, **Nettles** and **Thyme** are useful. **Antibacterial** herbs, **Yarrow**, **Liquorice** and **Basil** can be included and other **antiseptic** herbs that are easily available are **Fennel** and **Aniseed**.

C.O.P.D.
Chronic Obstructive Pulmonary Disease
(Heaves, Broken wind, Equine asthma, Hay fever, Allergies)

Probably the most common cause of chronic **coughing** in horses. This condition is caused by a horse developing a hypersensitivity to dust in the environment. Usually seen with the stabled horse where there may be poor ventilation, a dusty atmosphere or a mould may be present in poor quality hay or straw.

In summer months the problem can be encountered by horses that are outside. This is usually due to environmental reasons such as pollen from grass, agricultural crops or trees. In recent years the increasing growing of rape appears to have a significant adverse effect in both humans and horses causing a **hay fever** type condition.

Symptoms are usually a **cough** and a discharge of **mucus** and often pollen type **allergies** cause the eye to irritate and weep. There can also be an increase in the respiratory rate causing the horse to **heave**.

Temperature and **appetite** usually remain normal in horses suffering from **Chronic Obstructive Pulmonary Disease** although they are often lethargic. Initially the symptoms can be slight and they gradually worsen. Once a horse becomes susceptible to this problem it can re-occur very quickly and it has been likened to an **asthma** attack in humans.

The first action to take is to try to improve the environment that is causing the problem. Wood shavings, shredded paper or peat are all suitable replacements for straw bedding. Hay can be replaced with haylage or a cube alternative. Providing the horse is not affected by pollens, it is preferable to be kept at grass as much as possible.

A number of herbs can be helpful for both **Chronic Obstructive Pulmonary Disease** and less severe respiratory allergies. **Garlic** is probably the best known. **Aniseed, Liquorice, Thyme** and **Red Clover** are among those that can soothe and relax the respiratory system and help in the discharge of mucus.

PNEUMONIA

This is a severe respiratory condition that is caused by an infection in the lungs resulting from bacteria, **viral infection** or other foreign material being present such as **parasites**, or where a horse is **drenched** and the liquid goes down the wrong way.

In the case of **bacterial infections** or **viral infections** these can be highly contagious and horses can be infected through others **coughing**, therefore isolation is important.

Infection can also be spread by contact with infected tack or human contact, therefore extreme care should be taken. Not all **bacterial** or **viral infections** lead to pneumonia and early action can help in reducing the progression.

Infection is normally caused through inhalation although it can be transmitted in the **blood** of a newly born foal through the navel. Once infected **pus** and **inflammation** can form in the lungs, sometimes causing an **abscess** to develop.

Horses with pneumonia are very unwell and require immediate veterinary attention. There is a high temperature and an increased respiratory rate with **coughing** and a **nasal discharge**. The horse is dull and has no **appetite**.

Herbs with **expectorant** qualities such as **Marshmallow, Coltsfoot** and **Horehound** will help in the discharge of **mucus** and **pus** thus helping to clear the airways. Action also needs to be taken to reduce or kill the **bacterial infection**.

When a horse is recovering from pneumonia it should be encouraged to keep its head down to graze or eat. This improves the pathway for **mucus** to discharge through the nostrils and helps to clear the airways.

The prevention of pneumonia is of paramount importance. Boosting the **immune system** defence mechanism by feeding **Echinacea** is one way of helping in the fight against **bacteria** and **viral infections**.

PLEURISY
This is where there is **inflammation** of the membranes in the chest cavity and covering the lungs. Pleurisy is usually caused by a **bacterial infection** that can be secondary to **pneumonia**. Other factors such as severe **stress**, extreme climate changes or other infections can bring on this condition. The infection causes **pus** to increase in the chest cavity thus restricting expansion of the lungs and making breathing more difficult. Once the infection is in the bloodstream the horse deteriorates rapidly which makes this a source of great concern.

Veterinary attention is important. In many cases fluid may be removed from the chest cavity using a syringe. **This is a life threatening condition and needs immediate attention.**

THE CIRCULATORY SYSTEM

The Circulatory System	162
Blood	163
Anaemia	163
Hormonal System	163
Lymphangitis	164
Cushings Disease	165
Immune System	166

THE CIRCULATORY SYSTEM

The circulatory system is where the pumping of **blood** through arteries and veins acts as a carrier throughout the body. It carries oxygen from the lungs to muscles and tissues, and digested food from the gut to the **liver** and from there to other tissues. **Blood** also carries **hormones**, regulates the water and **electrolyte** balance and helps protect against infection by mobilising the bodies natural defences.

Any weakness or ailment of the circulatory system, through poor quality or an insufficient supply of **blood**, will have a profound effect and result in damage to the organs or tissues involved. It follows that disease in any organ may be caused as a result of a poor functioning **circulatory system** where either insufficient **blood** is supplied, or waste substances are not cleared away.

Where there is poor circulation there may be insufficient **blood** supply through the **kidneys** which can result in **fluid retention**. This may be apparent by a water build up resulting in **filled legs**. In such cases **diuretic** herbs can be useful. The best known and most suitable is **Dandelion**, since this herb also contains a high level of **potassium** which can be lost using other diuretics.

BLOOD
Blood is made up from **red and white cells** that are carried in fluid called **plasma**. **Plasma** contains over 90% of water, and about 6% **protein. Sodium, potassium, calcium, magnesium, chlorides,** bicarbonates and organic acid collectively account for about 1%.

Red cells give **blood** its colour. It is the **red cells** that transport oxygen from the lungs to the body tissues. They have a life of about 30 days and are then destroyed in the **spleen** and **liver**. They are replaced by new cells that are produced in the **bone marrow** normally at a rate to balance the cell numbers. It is when there is a shortfall in replacement cells that a horse becomes **anaemic**.

ANAEMIA
Anaemia can result in too many **red cells** being destroyed, or too few new cells being produced. A great number of illnesses and infections can cause this and it is important to establish what infection, **growth**, injury or ailment is causing the reduction in **red cells**.

Iron, vitamin B12 and **folic acid** are important in the production of **red cells**.

White cells destroy bacteria and play a fundamental role in the immunity of the body. They gather together where there is infection or damaged tissue and play a part in the **inflammatory** process.

THE HORMONAL SYSTEM
Glands control the hormonal status of the individual by producing **hormones** which are then carried in the bloodstream to control organs. It is possible to measure **hormones** in the bloodstream. However, this only determines the hormonal level whilst it is in transit. Of equal importance is the ability of target organs to respond. It is therefore the balance between **hormone** producing **glands** and the number of receptors functioning on the target organ that determine the true hormonal state.

For example, a **gland** may excrete a large amount of **hormones** into the bloodstream but if there are few receptors functioning at the target organ then the **hormones** can not be fully utilised. This is a simple outline of the very complicated process that controls the bodies hormonal state.

Hormone secreting glands include the **brain** which also controls the nervous system. The **ovary** and **uterus hormonal** secretions are, of course, the controlling influences of the **reproductive system** in the mare. Whilst the **hormones** from the **pituitary gland** stimulate follicle development, **ovulation** and milk secretion as well as promoting increased levels of **protein, fat**, sugar and water in the body.

The **pancreas** helps control **blood** sugar levels, whilst the **thyroid gland** secretions control the general metabolic rate.
A number of problems have been attributed to both **underactive thyroid function** (hypothyroidism) and **overactive thyroid function** (hyperthyroidism). It has been found that under activity can result when there is an **iodine** deficiency. **Seaweed** is rich in **iodine**, therefore, it can be a useful supplement in those cases. It follows that **Seaweed** should not be fed to the horse with an **overactive thyroid**. This condition can make the horse anxious and **hyperactive**, therefore, herbs like **Valerian, Nettles** and **Yarrow** would be of more benefit.

LYMPHANGITIS

In carrying out its function of removing excess fluid and debris from an inflamed area the **lymphatic system** has an important role in the repair of an injury. Where there is an infection this can spread to the lymphatic vessels causing them to become inflamed and limiting their ability to function correctly. This results in filling of the legs, usually hind, bringing about **lameness** and **pain**. This condition is known as **lymphangitis**. This is distinct from **filled legs** which is normally a management problem that may result from a horse standing in and can simply be resolved with exercise. Because it is infection from the wound area that has caused the spread into the **lymphatic** system, the first action required is to locate and treat the infected area.

Analgesics will help relieve **pain** which may enable the horse to be walked. Movement can be helpful in promoting circulation to the **lymph glands** and this helps restore its ability to reducing the filling.

Sometimes a pregnant mare will have a swelling on the belly where the **lymphatic system** becomes overburdened by the extra demands that the pregnancy brings. This usually disperses normally after foaling when the **lymphatic system** is able to cope with its work again.

Lymphatic "cleansing" herbs are **Cleavers, Marigold** and **Echinacea** and these can be combined to make a general tonic.

CUSHING'S DISEASE

Cushing's Disease has come to prominence more and more recently and it is increasingly being diagnosed, particularly in the U.S.A.

This is a condition that results from a **benign tumour** in the **pituitary gland** which is situated at the base of the brain. The function of the **pituitary gland** is adversely affected resulting in **hormonal** changes throughout the body.

Symptoms include a greater water intake with a corresponding increase in urinating, loss of condition and a long coat which encourages more **sweating**. Other symptoms can include skin infections or **abscesses**, even **laminitis** and **respiratory conditions** can result from this extremely unpleasant condition which is the cause of great concern to both horse owners and the veterinary profession. At present there seems to be no recognised cure although the herbal approach may help give some relief.

Red Clover and **Burdock Root** are reputed to have **anti-tumour** qualities and should be included in any herbal blend along with **Echinacea** to support the **immune system**. **Cleavers** and **Seaweed** will help maintain the **lymphatic system** whilst **Milk Thistle** is an excellent herb to support **liver** function. As always **Garlic** should be included for its all round beneficial qualities.

IMMUNE SYSTEM

The bodies own immune system gives it the ability to fight off illness or disease and it is when it is unable to cope with the task that infection takes over. The herbal approach to good health is to reduce the factors that have a negative effect and to enhance the immune system through good management and a balanced diet. External influences such as environmental pollutants are not always easy to avoid although the intake of synthetic substances and drugs can have an impact on the immune system and they are greatly over used. Internal influences such as **stress** and worry can have a weakening effect on the bodies natural defences and in the case of our horses, most of these are brought about by the way we keep them. A good balanced diet, exercise and plenty of fresh air are the first essentials in maintaining good health.

Herbs that help strengthen the immune system include **Echinacea, Red Clover** and **Garlic** whilst **Cleavers** and **Dandelion** will help in the process of **detoxifying**.

THE URINARY SYSTEM

The function of the urinary system is to maintain water and **electrolyte** balance and to excrete waste products.

Malfunction of the urinary system can be through **kidney**, urethra or **bladder infection.**

Horses usually urinate at rest. They can be very regular in their routine and often urinate when returning to their stall. It is quite common for a horse to grunt or groan when passing urine.

Adult horses urinate between four to six times daily depending on diet and water intake. When a mare is in **oestrus** her urine may be darker and more frequent than normal.

Signs of an infection or problem in the urinary system can be easily noticeable. Variations in the amount a horse urinates and stronger smelling urine are obvious signs of discomfort, as are straining or excessive groaning. The most common problems in the urinary system are minor infections or **chills**.

The **kidney** can continue to function in spite of considerable damage. Although there may be an injury or disease the **kidney** has the unusual ability to compensate making the symptoms uncommon. For this reason, by the time that **kidney** conditions are apparent they can be quite serious, often affecting other parts of the body.

Cystitis is inflammation of the bladder. It is not common in horses and as in humans, is more prevalent in females. Symptoms can include straining and more frequent attempts than normal to urinate. The urine can be discoloured by **blood**.

A blend of herbs that will act as an overall tonic for the **kidneys** and urinary system are **Horsetail, Parsley, Alfalfa, Strawberry** and **Golden Rod.**

Couch Grass and **Yarrow** are two herbs that are ideal for **cystitis**.

The best prevention for most conditions of the urinary system is to ensure that an adequate supply of fresh clean drinking water is always available.

THE COAT AND SKIN

The Coat and Skin	170
Sweet Itch	171
Allergic Reactions	172
Ringworm	172
Insect Bites	173
Lice	173
Dermatitis	174
Rain Scald	174
Cracked Heels (Mud Fever)	174
Growths	175
Melanomas	176
Warts	176
Sarcoids	177
Abscesses	177
Pigmentation	178
Wounds	178

THE COAT AND SKIN

The coat and skin are much more than a visible sheath over the body. They have many functions including helping to control body temperature. In cold climates long hair is produced to increase insulation. Once the hair grows, the follicles then rest until long daylight hours stimulate new hair growth which pushes out the old hairs and produce the summer coat. This process continues thereby renewing all hair throughout the year. The exceptions to this are the tail and mane, which continue to grow for several years.

Regular grooming will not only remove surface dirt and loose hairs but the brushing action helps to stimulate bloodflow and tone the muscles. It will also help to recognise if there are any irregularities or blemishes in the skin and in the early detection of problems. The condition of coat and skin can mirror the well being of the horse.

Both can be greatly affected by internal and external factors such as **liver** disease, **malignant tumours** and **photosensitisation** and they are a good indication of poor health. External influences such as environment, **insect infestation** and **ring worm** can cause irritable reactions that may result in local **hair loss**.

Another benefit from the daily routine of grooming a horse is that the direct contact between handler and animal can help in building a trusting relationship.

SKIN ALLERGIES

SWEET ITCH

This is an **allergic reaction** to the **bites** of **midges**. It is most common in ponies although all types of horses can be affected. This is a seasonal problem. **Midges** are active from April to November. They mostly bite at daybreak and nightfall in humid climates. **Midges** are more prevalent in wooded and lake-land areas. The worst affected areas are usually where the long hair is; mane, tail base, forelock etc. and the resulting irritation causes horses to scratch and rub against any surface, rubbing away hair and often making the areas very sore. Once a horse or pony has suffered with sweet itch it usually re-occurs each season. Good management can help in preventing or reducing the extent of the problem. Where possible the horse should be stabled or kept away from vulnerable areas during daybreak and nightfall.

Herbs can be very helpful in the prevention of sweet itch. The most common used being **Garlic**. Many people add **Garlic** to the daily feed continuously and one of its many benefits are its **diaphoretic** qualities. Once the **Garlic** is in the system it excretes through the skin of the horse and makes it an unappetising surface for **midges** and **flies**. By taking early preventative action it is possible to prevent sweet itch getting started. However when feeding **Garlic** it is most important to ensure that the product you buy is pure **Garlic**. Many so called **Garlic** powders on the market are filled out with other substances such as lime stone flour. We always use pure **Garlic** granules and have found them both effective and pleasant to use. Where sweet itch has already started it is likely that more than **Garlic** will be needed. **Alterative** herbs such as **Cleavers** are good. Also **Nettles, Seaweed** and **Burdock** are other herbs that would combine well to help with this problem. **Echinacea** is another possible addition to help build up the **immune system** in horses that are badly affected.

We have found that the best way of dealing with sweet itch is from the inside and feeding herbs can be extremely effective. In cases where the skin is severely rubbed and sore the healing process can be expedited by applying **Tea Tree** cream.

ALLERGIC REACTIONS (HIVES, NETTLE RASH)

Allergic reactions to the **skin** may result from **insect bites**. A reaction to something eaten, injection of drugs or contact with some infectious disease.

Occasionally a horse will have an **allergic reaction** to **proteins** in feeds or even fresh grass at certain times. Such allergies normally produce small lumps over the surface of the **skin** and can be the result of excessive feeding of **protein** in relation to the exercise being given. This is because the food upsets the **protein** and **electrolyte** balance and the **lymph glands** are unable to carry away the excess waste material and fluid. Such cases also often result in **filled legs.**

Circulation can be improved by using **alterative** herbs such as those used for **sweet itch** with the addition of **Dandelion** which acts as a **diuretic** and where there is severe infection **Echinacea** should be added.

RINGWORM

Contrary to some beliefs ringworm is not caused by a worm. It is a highly contagious **fungal infection**, which can be picked up from stable surfaces, tack and other animals. The problem with ringworm is that the fungi can survive for a year or so, thus causing an infection in other horses sometime after it appears to have cleared up. For example, where a rug has been used on a horse suffering from ringworm it may harbour the infection and reappear next time the rug is used. The movement of horses to sales, shows and the use of infected tack from horse to horse can make ringworm a big problem in racing or competition yards.

It is usually apparent within a week or two of contact for the signs to be noticeable. Small circular areas of infection appear on the **skin**. Although they do not normally cause itchiness, the hair gradually falls out on the affected areas leaving the **skin** scaly.

It is worth mentioning that humans and other animals can also be infected with, and can spread ringworm. Therefore, proper precautions should be taken when grooming or treating an infected horse.

Tea Tree cream is a very good **antifungal** and it can be applied externally on the affected areas. It will not only help combat local infection but also in repairing damaged **skin**.

Bad cases of ringworm can make a horse very poorly making further treatment necessary. **Alterative** herbs such as **Cleavers** and **Burdock** together with **Garlic** can be fed along with **Echinacea** to help fight infection.

INSECT BITES

Feeding **Garlic** can be a good deterrent to insects since once in the system the natural insect repelling **sulphur** is excreted through the **skin**. This makes for an unappetising landing site for **flies, ticks** and other insects. Also **Garlic** juice can be applied externally where its **antiseptic** qualities will help soothe and heal whilst simultaneously acting as a repellent.

External application of **Tea Tree** cream can help soothe and heal **insect bites**.

LICE

Lice are six legged flat insects with no wings. There are two species and they will both spend their entire lives of about three weeks on the surface of a horses **skin** . One is blood sucking whilst the other **bites**.

Lice attach eggs (**nits**) usually in the long hair parts and young lice emerge from them in about 10 days. They can be passed by direct contact from horse to horse and even by rugs, tack and other equipment.

This condition is usually found in poorly kept horses that are out on pasture receiving little attention. The **coat** has flaky **skin** debris resulting from the actions of the lice and is often damaged by the horse rubbing or biting the irritating areas.

Horses who are daily groomed would not be troubled by lice.

Treatment is often by completely spraying or dusting the area with a propriety product containing insecticides but a wash using dilute **Tea Tree** oil offers a more natural effective cure with the added advantage that it will help against infection and heal the **skin**.

The best prevention for lice is to add **Garlic** to the feed and groom daily.

DERMATITIS
This is normally a seasonal condition that is an **allergic reaction** to insects – see **sweet itch**.

However, there are other conditions that will adversely affect the **skin** and cause dermatitis. For example some chemicals and detergents will cause an irritation to the **skin** and can result in **inflammation** and soreness, in extreme cases even loss of **skin**! The obvious answer to these problems is to immediately stop applying any substance that causes a **skin** reaction and to wash off the area with warm water.

Tea Tree cream can be applied externally. Where infection has taken place, **Echinacea** should be fed with **Seaweed** which is rich in **iodine**.

RAIN SCALD, CRACKED HEELS, MUD FEVER, SCRATCHES (U.S.A.)
Rain scald, cracked heels, mud fever and scratches all relate to the same condition which is caused by an organism which gains entry into the **skin** when it is saturated.

Because this condition is associated with wet conditions it normally affects horses that are turned out. However, it can also affect stabled horses particularly when they are on deep litter.

The incidence of rain scald or cracked heel is higher in horses with a lot of hair due to the excessive moisture retained which causes prolonged wetness of **skin**, thus increasing the likelihood of damage and irritation by mud. Some horses seem more prone to this condition such as those with white socks and sensitive **skin**. Poor hygiene and a failure to treat this condition early can result in secondary infection. The classic case of rain scald, cracked heels or mud fever show signs of **inflammation** and soreness. With mud fever there are often cracks in the **skin** at the back of the pastern hence the name cracked heel.

This soreness causes pain and in severe cases **lameness**. Infection results from bacterial attack in the open wound.

Good management will help prevent or reduce the incidence of rain scald and cracked heels. Cleaning and drying after exercise is most important and it will usually prevent the problem starting. Where there is already infection it is important to scrub clean all external parts and dry thoroughly. Usually a good **Tea Tree** cream can be applied externally and this will help against infection and the re-growth of damaged **skin**.

Echinacea can be fed to help build up the body's resistance in the fight against infection.

As with most **skin** infections, **alterative** herbs such as **Cleavers** can help in "cleansing" the system.

GROWTHS

The terms **tumour, growth, cancer** or **cyst** are all used to describe an abnormal growth that causes swelling. Where the growth is restricted it is normally referred to as **benign** whereas those that continue to produce new growth are regarded as invasive and referred to as **malignant**. The term cancer is usually applied to this type of growth.

Malignant growths can spread through the bloodstream as well as by invading local tissue. They are very serious and require specialist attention that may involve surgery and radioactive treatment. Scientists continue to discover new properties in herbs that may help in the treatment of cancer. **Red Clover** is one of a number of herbs that are reputed to be of benefit. Probably the best single herb to help support the **immune system** is **Echinacea**.

MELANOMA

A melanoma is a **benign tumour** that affects the **skin**. There seems to be a higher incidence of melanomas in grey horses. These unpleasant lumps often occur inside the back legs or under the tail and they can be a particular nuisance to the nursing mare. They can also affect any other part of the body and sometimes occur on the head.

When rubbed they get very sore and can become open to infection. Therefore, any herbal approach should include herbs to strengthen the **immune system** and combat infection.

Sometimes surgical removal of melanomas may be carried out. An old farmers method that has been used successfully is to place a small tight elastic band over the lump nearest to the **skin**. This gradually cuts off the **blood** supply to the melanoma and it usually dies and falls off after about 3-4 weeks. The small resulting wound can be treated with **Tea Tree** cream and it should heal completely.

If feeding herbs, a combination of **Garlic, Seaweed, Fenugreek, Red Clover** and **Echinacea** would be a suitable blend. **Cleavers** can be added as an **alterative**.

WARTS

Warts are the most common type of **growth** in horses. It is usually young horses who are affected by warts, often from a dam to her foal. They can also pick up the **virus** from the stable or other surfaces that can help in the transmission from one horse to another. Warts are usually on the muzzle, nostrils or eyelids and other less hairy parts.

Often multiple, these unpleasant grey lumps can be damaged causing them to bleed and making them open to secondary infection. The so called milk warts that appear around the muzzle can disappear spontaneously after a couple of months.

The "old wives tale" of applying the pressed juice from **Dandelion** leaves or stalks appears to have some merit when applied on a regular basis.

External application of **Tea Tree** cream can reduce the incidence of infection. Some believe that a deficiency of **iodine** is a factor in warts and **Seaweed** can be fed to increase this. Feeding **Echinacea** will help build up the bodies **immune system** in its fight against secondary infection that can result from bleeding or open warts.

SARCOIDS (Angleberry)

Sarcoids are due to a different kind of **virus** to **warts** and they usually affect adult horses. They are a common **skin tumour** problem in a horse although they have the characteristics of a **benign tumour** they also demonstrate **malignant** properties by invading the **skin** and growing rapidly. Often sarcoids will grow on the inside of the thighs Unlike **warts,** they do not regress with age and the treatment is often to surgically remove them. However this does not always prevent them from returning. (see **growths**).

ABSCESSES

Abscesses result from a bacterial attack to a vulnerable area causing **infection** and **inflammation**.

Bacteria can affect internal organs such as the **digestive system** and lungs through ingesting and inhaling. It can also cause dental disease and penetrate body tissue through broken **skin**. The resulting **pus** becomes **poisonous** and infection will circulate throughout the body if it is not removed. **Strangles** (streptococcus equi infection) is a disease of the upper respiratory tract that normally affects young horses. The symptoms include a poor **appetite, fever** and **nasal discharge** with an abscess in the region of the **lymph glands**.

The **pus** from the abscess will spread the disease and complete isolation of the horse is necessary for this extremely infectious disease.

An added problem is that the **inflammation** that results from the infection can cause obstruction that inhibits the removal of **pus**. In such cases surgical removal may be necessary.

All abscesses are serious and many of the conditions can be contagious. It is therefore necessary to contact a veterinary surgeon immediately. In the case of minor abscesses that are readily accessible, such as in the **hoof**, it is normally possible to apply an external **poultice** to draw out the infection. In more severe cases a skilled farrier may be able to assist under veterinary supervision.

To help in the fight against infection **Fenugreek** and **Garlic** can be fed. **Antibacterial** herbs **Yarrow, Marigold** and **Echinacea** together with **Meadowsweet** that has **anti-inflammatory, antiseptic** and **alterative** qualities make a good blend.

PIGMENTATION
The general health of the horse can be reflected in the quality and condition of the **skin**. Likewise deficiencies of **vitamins** and **minerals** often result in poor pigmentation. An excellent herb to help restore good pigmentation is **Seaweed**.

WOUNDS
An open wound is where there is **skin** damage. The resulting bleeding depends on the severity of the damage but in all cases this needs to be minimised. Simple straight cuts usually bleed freely and are the quickest to heal. In many cases straightforward first aid procedures are sufficient for small cuts but whenever there is any doubt a veterinary surgeon should be called as soon as the bleeding is controlled.

Irregular cuts or tears, such as when a horse catches itself on barbed wire, can result in flaps of **skin** that are likely to gradually die. Sometimes parts can be **sutured** successfully if only to cover an open wound long enough to curtail infection.

More serious wounds are deeper ones that may not look bad but can do greater internal damage through penetrating soft tissue. A puncture from a stake or fork could cause such a wound. These, together with wounds that penetrate into the body cavities such as the abdomen, should always receive the urgent attention of a veterinary surgeon.

The best known healing herb is **Comfrey** and this can be fed in herb form or applied as a cream externally to the wound. Either way the use of **Comfrey** is likely to reduce the healing time. Where applied externally it will help reduce the incidence of proud flesh. However, it is important to ensure that a wound is completely free of infection before applying **Comfrey** cream externally since it is likely to promote healing of the outside tissue that it is in contact with before the inside.

Abrasions are often superficial and these can usually be successfully dealt with by applying normal first aid procedures.

Once correct diagnosis and initial treatment is carried out by the veterinary surgeon it is often possible to include herbal products into the repair and recovery programme. For example, simple abrasions and cuts will heal much quicker if a **Comfrey** cream is applied.

A closed wound is where the **skin** is not broken such as a **bruise, sprain, muscle, ligament** or **tendon** damage.

An **oedema** is where there is a soft swelling beneath the **skin** resulting from internal damage or disease and the cause of this should be investigated by the veterinary surgeon.

THE MUSCULAR AND SKELETAL SYSTEM

Arthritis and Rheumatism	182
Azoturia	183
Muscle Sprains	184
Tendon and Ligament Damage	185
Laminitis	186
Navicular Syndrome	187
Hoof Problems	187
Bruised Sole, Sore Feet	188
Bruising	189
Thrush	189
Fractures	190
Inflammation	191
Pain Relief	191

ARTHRITIS AND RHEUMATISM

Arthritis and **rheumatism** result from a friction between body parts of varying degrees. The herbal approach does not differentiate between these conditions.

Abnormal stresses on body parts can cause the breakdown of joints, cartilage and damage to the soft tissue structures which result in **inflammation** and restricted movement. These stresses can be brought about by conformational abnormalities which increase the stress on a joint. Injury or wear and tear can cause similar damage.

Arthritis is known as **Degenerative Joint Disease** (**D.J.D.**) which implies that this condition is regarded as irreversible and potentially progressive. Although it is normally associated with older horses, younger race or competition horses can suffer as a result of the severe stress, particularly to the lower limb joints.

Signs of arthritis and rheumatism are usually restricted movement or **lameness** and a veterinary examination should always be carried out. Sometimes local anaesthetics are used to establish the source of **pain** and x-rays can detect where there are resulting bone changes.

Rest will help with reducing **inflammation** in soft tissue but this usually returns with exercise. It is therefore normal for **anti-inflammatory** and **analgesics** to be used to enable the horse to maintain movement without being in **pain**. Such treatment is not effecting a cure, but is reducing the **pain** to improve movement. Controlled movement may bring about a fusion of the damaged parts leading to a reduction in **pain** from the affected area. There are a great number of herbs that can be beneficial for arthritis and rheumatism which should be treated as a whole with good management and diet. A good quality of life can be enjoyed and many horses are able to continue in their particular discipline. Indeed, in most cases regular exercise helps to maintain good circulation to the affected parts.

It depends on the severity of the problem as to what herbs might be best to feed. For example **Devils Claw** is an extremely good **anti-inflammatory** and **analgesic** herb, but it will do little other than reducing **inflammation** and **pain**. Where a horse has been condemned to long term use of **pain** killing drugs **Devils Claw** is usually a good alternative. However it is our preference to include other herbs where possible so as to help the condition rather than just remove **pain**. **Willow** and **Meadowsweet** are herbs that can also be helpful. They contain **salicilic acid** which makes them similar in action to Aspirin.

Any aid to improving **blood** circulation is desirable. **Nettles** and **Dandelion** are among those that have that function as well as being rich in **iron** and **vitamin C**. Damaged bone or tissue can be helped by feeding **Comfrey** which will quicken the fusing and repair process. **Cider Apple Vinegar** is an old remedy used by farmers and this can be added to either food or water. Some companies dilute **Cider Apple Vinegar** which reduces the effectiveness and the best yardstick is the acidity levels, which should be over 5%.

AZOTURIA
(Tying Up, Set Fast)

Azoturia is a poorly understood condition that results in muscle damage. The symptoms are typically stiffness that occurs soon after the start of exercise. This condition is normally associated with fit racehorses or eventers who are being fed high concentrated feed. The stiffness of the back and hindquarters causes **pain** and a reluctance to move. In severe cases **sweating** takes place as a reaction to the **pain**. The exact cause is not known, although **stress** and exercise seem to play their part. A deficiency of **vitamin E, selenium, sodium, potassium** and **calcium** have all been said to be significant factors. The relationship between diet and exercise is an important one and the horse should not be fed in anticipation of an increase in work. It is better to wait until additional energy is required before increasing the intake. It follows that if a horse has a day off then concentrate feed should be reduced.

Simply reducing **protein** by substituting bran in itself is not ideal because this can cause a **calcium/phosphorus** imbalance. A good balanced proprietary ration is usually suitable with the addition of salt to promote drinking of fresh water.

The incidence of azoturia seems to be greater in mares and it may be that the **hormonal changes** throughout the spring and summer months have an effect on this.

Herbs that are rich in the deficient **vitamins** and **minerals** are **Fenugreek, Seaweed, Meadowsweet, Dandelion** and **Nettles**. A combination of these have proved to be of great benefit to horses suffering with azoturia. It is important to maintain body salts and **electrolytes** should be used after exercise where necessary.

MUSCLE SPRAINS

Muscular sprains and damage are inevitable in active and competition horses who are under constant tension and pressure. As in humans, damage can result from an insufficient warm up period before undertaking strenuous exercise. Poor conformation can increase the likelihood of sprains and a skilful farrier who prepares correctly shaped, well balanced feet can contribute by helping overcome minor conformational defects that could create undue tension or strain on muscles. Poor fitting tack can also cause muscle problems and even poor riding will unbalance the horse and increase the risk of damage.

The consequence of muscle sprains or damage can be **pain** and **inflammation** and there are a number of ways of reducing these through both internal and external means. Depending on the position of the injury cold hosing can be soothing. The application of a tincture or cream of **Arnica** can "bring out" the bruising.

Massage and also muscle manipulation can stimulate healing and be of particular benefit in the back region (see **McTimoney chiropractic**).

Herbs will help in repairing damage and reducing **pain** (see **tendon** and **ligament** damage).

TENDON AND LIGAMENT DAMAGE

A blow or strain causing damage to tendons or ligaments probably accounts for more time lost in race and competition horses than any other. From a minor sprain through to being completely broken down the requirement is nearly always the same: time to allow the bodies own systems to set about the natural healing process.

By way of first aid the injured area should be hosed down with cold water and where possible supported with correct bandaging using gauzes to maintain even support. In all cases the opposite leg should be supported since it may come under more strain whilst the injured one is rested. The over tightening of bandages can do more harm so it is important that this task is carried out by an experienced horse person.

The next thing to do is to establish the exact nature and extent of the injury. In some cases this may require the use of diagnostic ultrasound equipment. This is similar to that used for pregnancy tests and it provides the veterinary surgeon with a detailed scan of the test area.

Usually a period of **box rest** is required when initial treatment may include an **anti-inflammatory** and **analgesic**. Often a drug such as **phenylbutazone** is prescribed for this purpose. There are herbs that have similar qualities, such as **Devils Claw** and some veterinary surgeons would be willing to use this since it will not slow down the healing process in the way that the drug might.

One herb that is sure to help the healing process is **Comfrey**. Traditionally known as **knitbone** this herb can be just as effective in the healing of tissue as it is bone and can be fed daily in conjunction with other treatments.

Other herbs that are suitable in helping in the repair of sprains and more serious damage include those that will promote bloodflow and aid the **lymphatic system**. A blend of **Burdock, Celery, Dandelion, Golden Rod, Nettles** and **Seaweed** would be a good general mix for this purpose. Where a horse has to stand in for some time he may benefit from relaxing herbs (see **Box Rest**).

LAMINITIS
Founders

This is an unpleasant condition that can take some time to relieve. It is where the sensitive laminae of the foot becomes inflamed through an insufficient **blood** supply resulting in a lack of nutrients to the cells causing damage and **inflammation**. The hard hoof covering of the foot restricts the space for swelling and increases pressure and **pain** in the foot. Laminitis usually affects overweight horses and ponies that are turned out when the grass is rich and fast growing. It can also be caused by excessive **carbohydrates** in hard feed or through a trauma to the **digestive system**. It is an "overload" of the **digestive system** that results in acid conditions in the gut which kill off natural bacteria and allows the release of **toxins** into the system to adversely affect the **blood** flow throughout the body including the capillaries to the feet. There are other conditions that can release **toxins** into the bloodstream such as infection caused through a mare aborting and this can result in laminitis, as can damage caused through continual work on hard ground.

In all cases the treatment needs to help relieve **pain** and stimulate **blood** flow. A restricted diet is the first step when it is apparent that a horse has been over-consuming. A limited area or even box confinement may be necessary. It is helpful to maintain some movement where possible to promote **blood** flow so where box confinement is required some in hand exercise may be appropriate. Some relief can be gained by trimming by an experienced farrier and in extreme cases a veterinary surgeon may remove some of the outer horn.

Devils Claw will help reduce **inflammation** and relieve **pain**. **Willow** has similar qualities as well as thinning the **blood**. Herbs such as **Nettles, Cleavers** and **Garlic** will assist with circulation. **Seaweed** and **Rosehips** will help in the re-growth of horn.

It is important to ensure that a reduced diet does not bring about a deficiency in **vitamins** and **minerals**. Specialist herbal suppliers can advise on how herbs can help and most good feed companies can offer nutritional advice and a range of suitable high fibre feeds.

NAVICULAR SYNDROME

This disease relates to the area of the navicular bone which is situated behind the pedal bone in the foot. It normally only affects the front feet of horses and rarely affects ponies.

It is generally believed that a major cause of navicular disease is an impaired **blood** flow to the back of the foot. This may result from poor **circulation** through **blood** clots or a thickening of the artery walls. This can be a painful disease that results in a shortening of stride and lameness, particularly on hard ground.

Much can be done to help this condition by a good farrier by correctly trimming and balancing the foot so that it stands squarely on the ground. Normally the toe is kept short and this helps to encourage the growth of the heel. A flat shoe is often fitted that will allow for expansion at the heel.

Circulation is very important and where possible an exercise routine should be maintained. This will encourage normal **blood** flow. Movement can also be maintained by daily turnout in a paddock. There are a number of herbs that can help with this condition. **Meadowsweet** and **Willow** help thin the blood whilst **Devils Claw** will help reduce **pain** and swelling. **Nettles** are good for circulation as is **Cider Apple Vinegar**.

HOOF PROBLEMS

Horses in the wild do not have the regular attention of a farrier. It takes from 8 to 12 months for new horn to grow from the coronary band to the foot edge. This rate would compensate for normal wear in a natural environment. Growth varies according to diet and often poor condition of the horn is a reflection of the overall condition of a horse.

Because horses are rarely in the natural environment we have to consider the wear that results from the additional work that we give them. Shoes were introduced to enable horses to travel many miles over hard surfaces without resulting in undue wear to the foot.

When you consider the bulk of the horses weight is carried by the hoof wall, with some weight taken by the frog, it can be appreciated the need to maintain a healthy foot. The horn is very similar to our finger or toe nails in that it is not sensitive and it continues to grow. An incorrectly balanced foot in the horse can result in strain or damage to other parts therefore it is essential that hooves are correctly trimmed and balanced at least once a month. Indeed, corrective trimming by a skillful farrier can ensure that feet are shaped to encourage the formation of straight limbs.

It has been said that black horn is stronger than white. However, the colour is purely due to pigment granules that may reduce the rate of wear but they do not affect the strength. Heavy or wet surfaces can soften the hoof causing it to wear down quicker than on drier surfaces.

The foot is designed to prevent the weight being carried on the sole of the foot. Where the edge of a foot is worn down or over-trimmed the effect would be similar to dropped soles which make them more liable to **bruising** and **lameness**.

The application of external hoof oils is of questionable benefit to the health of the foot. Keeping the foot cleaned out and free from damp bedding is of more importance. External massaging of the coronary band can assist in promoting **blood** flow and growth. **Blood** flow to the foot can also be improved by feeding herbs such as **Nettles** and **Cleavers** which together with **Seaweed** and **Rosehips** are rich in **calcium** and **vitamin C** and will help promote **hoof** growth.

BRUISED SOLE, SORE FEET

Flat footed horses are more prone to bruised sole which can result from standing on a stone, a poor fitting shoe, or continuous work on hard ground. The signs can be immediate, such as when a horse steps on a stone, or less pronounced when sore feet may cause a pottery or restricted movement.

Once the problem is correctly diagnosed poulticing the foot is usually helpful. In many cases the removal of the shoe is necessary particularly where they are ill fitting. A good farrier can be a great help in both locating the problem and trimming a foot to help relieve pain.

As in general bruising, the external application of **Arnica** cream or tincture can be beneficial as can the application of **Witch Hazel**. Depending upon the severity of the swelling **anti-inflammatory** herbs can be fed together with **Comfrey** to help repair any damage.

BRUISING

Bruising is usually the result of damage to tissue through a kick, fall or other injury and is common among competitive horses. The swollen area often causes **lameness**, which varies according to location and severity.

For external bruising to the leg, shoulder or to other muscular areas the external application of **Arnica** cream or tincture is extremely helpful. **Anti-inflammatory** herbs can be fed to reduce swelling and **Comfrey** will help expedite healing to damaged tissue.

Mares often have bruising of the vaginal area as a result of a large or difficult **foaling**. Usually in these cases the mare will be examined fully to ensure there is no other post foaling injury.

Great care is necessary in applying cream around the vaginal area and as always veterinary advice should be sought (see **Foaling**).

THRUSH

Thrush results from moist material causing infection in the frog cleft. Where it remains untreated it can progress into the sensitive tissue of the foot causing **lameness**. Thrush is caused by a failure to clean the feet correctly and by allowing a horse to stand on dirty bedding.

This is a condition that can be prevented by good management and hygiene. Feet should be cleaned properly on a daily basis and a good clean dry bed should be maintained for the horse to stand on.

When treatment is required it may be necessary for a farrier to trim and remove the infected part of the frog and the foot should be thoroughly scrubbed using a diluted salt and **Tea Tree** solution. Where there has been infection, **Echinacea** can be fed to help build the bodies own defences.

FRACTURES

Fractures are usually the result of direct trauma and they range from difficult to impossible to treat in a horse. The severity and location of damage as well as the size and temperament of the horse are important factors as to the outcome. A simple fracture, where a bone breaks in two pieces but remains in place, may be able to be supported whilst it repairs. If a bone breaks through the surrounding tissue and skin it becomes a compound fracture and there is increased risk of infection. The prospect of repair through surgery brings the additional risk associated with the recovery from general anaesthetic.

Unlike humans, you can not tell a horse to lie down and stay still. Their natural instinct to stand and run not only hinders the repairing process but can also do more damage.

Where a fracture is not clearly identifiable through examination, x-rays will be taken. In some cases the fracture can be almost indetectable and it may be necessary for further x-rays to be taken a week or so later when the healing process makes it easier to identify the damaged area.

It is necessary to restrict movement and where **box rest** is required **sedative** or **relaxing herbs** may help. Painkillers are used carefully to ensure that the horse does not over use the damaged limb. It is necessary to do all that is possible to help in the repair of the bone and providing this remains in line a bony callus will form to re-unite the two pieces. Once the healing is completed the callus join is still detectable but reduces in size. The best herb for dealing with fractures is **Comfrey**. This can be added to the daily feed up to the rate of 50 gms per day and will help speed up the healing process in both bone and tissue.

We have experienced incredible results after feeding **Comfrey** for just two or three weeks.

Wherever there has been damage, especially in joints, there is an increased likelihood of subsequent **arthritis** and consideration needs to be given to herbs that can help with this condition.

INFLAMMATION

Inflammation is a response to infection or injury. It is characterised by redness, swelling, heat and **pain** and results in a loss of function.

The extent of swelling is usually an indication of the severity of the infection or injury and the cause needs to be established before undertaking treatment. In many cases this may be due to a blow or strain and the inflammation process becomes apparent immediately. In others it may be a gradual process caused through infection or disease.

Once the cause of inflammation has been established it may be appropriate to consider feeding **anti-inflammatory** herbs together with others to help in repair and healing. Some herbs will also act as **analgesics** and may not be appropriate in all cases since they may encourage a horse to over-use a damaged limb.

PAIN RELIEF

Pain is the common symptom of many injuries, diseases and other conditions and in many cases it is the one that manifests the problem. For example, if a horse is lame in one leg then it is almost certainly a reaction to pain. Such obvious signs are helpful in diagnosing the problem since before a veterinary surgeon can accurately treat a horse he needs to identify both the source and the underlying cause of the condition. Often **inflammation** is associated with pain and that may be more apparent to the observer than the pain itself.

There are a number of herbs that have **analgesic** qualities often combined with other characteristics such as in the case of **Devils Claw** which is also **anti-inflammatory**. Reducing pain in itself may not be the correct path to restoring good health and an overview of the situation needs to be taken by the prescribing veterinary surgeon. Where it is appropriate **Devils Claw** can play a valuable part since it works in harmony with the other functions of the body and will not impede the normal healing process.

THE REPRODUCTIVE SYSTEM

The Oestrus Cycle	194
Pregnancy	195
Foaling	196
Foal Scour	197
Mastitis	198
Milk Production	199
Fertility	199
Rigs or False Rigs	201

THE OESTRUS CYCLE

The oestrus cycle usually lasts twenty-one days. Five days of **oestrus** (in season) and sixteen days of **dioestrus** when a mare is not receptive to a stallion. Normally a mare cycles during spring and summer, which is normally regarded as the breeding season. She ceases to cycle (becomes **anoestrus**) throughout the autumn and winter months.

A filly will start to cycle during her second year and continue throughout her life.

The oestrus cycle brings about **hormonal changes** that are designed to enable the mare to conceive if covered by a stallion at the correct time. These **hormonal changes** are a necessary part of the reproductive system in the mare.

Throughout the oestrus cycle a change in the behaviour of a mare is usually noticeable. This behaviour change reflects at what stage of the cycle the mare is at, and her ability to conceive. For example, a mare running loose with a stallion will ensure that the male advances are rebuffed when she is **dioestrus**, whereas when she is **oestrus** (in season) she will gradually warm to the approaches made. This is nature's way of ensuring that a mare is only covered at the time when she is likely to conceive.

The days just before **oestrus** are the times when a mare might be less amenable. These **hormonal** changes can make the mare very uncomfortable and irritable. **PMT (PMS)** behaviour is common and results in some mares being very aggressive. Thankfully such behaviour usually only lasts a few days and is soon forgotten – until next time round!

There are a number of herbs that can help with the **hormonal changes** and the discomfort that can result, as well as general **calming** and **relaxing** herbs.

Chaste Tree is a well known herb for **PMT (PMS)** type behaviour and is renowned for helping hormonal disorders. **Valerian Root** has similar benefits as well as having **sedative** and **relaxing** qualities.

Other herbs that would complement each other to make a suitable blend include **Chamomile** and **Dandelion**.

It is not always easy to identify the oestrus cycle in a mare – some seem to be "mareish" most of the time. Equally it can seem as though a mare is permanently in season throughout the spring and summer where she continuously displays an unusual behaviour pattern. Both of these situations can be due to a **hormonal change** and herbs can be helpful in controlling this behaviour.

There are drugs that are used for inducing or controlling the oestrus cycle. These are used under veterinary control usually for the purpose of preparing a mare, for covering and maximising the chances of conception (see **fertility**).

PREGNANCY

Pregnancy in a thoroughbred mare is approximately eleven months. This varies in different breeds with ponies and small breeds being shorter by anything up to 3 weeks. Nowadays it is possible to detect pregnancy at a very early stage through ultrasound scanning, and professional studs routinely check mares sometimes as early as 14 days after covering. At such an early stage it is not possible to detect twin pregnancies, therefore a second scan is usually taken a few days after and a final scan at about 42 days. It is extremely unusual for a mare to carry twins full term and if no preventative action is taken in the case of twinning the pregnancy may absorb, or the mare abort at a later stage.

Once a mare is checked in foal and it is established that there is only one foetus, the mare can be treated normally. She should be fed with a good balanced diet and kept in good all round condition. Do not overfeed a pregnant mare, particularly early on.

The last quarter of the pregnancy is when the foal increases its size five fold and it is in the last weeks that special attention needs to be paid to the diet and condition of the mare. As the pregnancy advances and the foetus grows the mare becomes more uncomfortable. It is better to feed little and often, say four times daily, so as to help avoid the discomfort of large amounts of food in the **digestive system**.

It is not uncommon during late pregnancy for a mare to have a swelling on the belly. This is due to the additional load on the **lymphatic system** and usually causes no problem.

Herbs can be extremely beneficial to the foaling mare – but they can also be harmful. Therefore, it is important that you pay special attention to which herbs are most suited (see also **foaling**).

FOALING

The foaling of a mare can be one of the most satisfying experiences, or one of the worst!

In their natural environment most mares will foal and cleanse without a problem and the foal will be up and moving often within minutes. Our "domestication" and interference in the natural habitat and breeding of horses has had an effect on their foaling. The more structured management which often includes stabling, limited exercise and a controlled diet all have an effect on the in-foal mare and her behaviour.

Over 90% of mares would probably foal successfully unattended resulting in a live foal. However, because of the frequent interference in the management of a pregnancy it is necessary for a qualified person to be in attendance. For example, in the case of thoroughbred breeding it is not uncommon for a mare to be stitched after covering. In such cases the stud groom, or vet, would normally have to cut the mare just before foaling to avoid her tearing and doing more damage to herself. This process of stitching and then cutting is one that we believe may be too commonly used, but it is justified as being a means of reducing the incidence of infection in the early **pregnancy** thus maximising the chances of success.

In all cases it is desirable for an experienced person to be in attendance at the time a mare is due to foal. Like so many things the important thing about **foaling** is knowing what is normal and what is not. When something is wrong there should be somebody that recognises there is a problem and is able to deal with it. To telephone a vet during a foaling that is problematical may be too late because things happen quickly once the foaling process starts.

There is much that can be said on the subject of foaling but space does not permit that here. The over riding message, as always, is to have an expert in attendance when required.

From a dietary point of view there are a number of herbs that can be of assistance to the foaling mare of which **Raspberry** is probably the best known. These will help in relaxing the pelvic muscles and the foaling and cleansing process. Other herbs such as **Fenugreek** will promote milk flow and of course **Echinacea** will help ensure that the **immune system** is more able to deal with any infection. Also **Seaweed**, **Nettles, Chamomile** and **Garlic** all combine to make an excellent blend suitable for the foaling mare.

Generally speaking it is only necessary to feed these herbs for about one month before, and after foaling. There are some herbs that should be avoided when feeding a pregnant mare since they can act as a **uterine stimulant** and bring about premature foaling. An example is **Devils Claw**. It is therefore important that when feeding herbs to a pregnant mare you ensure they are safe and suitable for that purpose.

FOAL SCOUR

This is common in foals when they are about 10 days old, at the time when the mare has her **foaling heat**. Scouring can be caused by digestive upset through nutrition or through **worms**. It was always believed that the changes in the mares milk when she came into **foaling heat** caused it to become richer and the foal scouring resulted from the nutritional changes. However, recent opinion is that the scouring is as a result of **threadworm**. The infection is passed in the mares milk when the foal is only a few days old and the rapidly developing eggs will be passed through the foals **digestive system** and in its faeces by the time that the foal is 10 days old. The eggs can develop and multiply further outside producing an increase of larvae that could re-infect the foal. As in all cases of **worms**, preventative action can help and a good worming programme in the mare is important. **Garlic** is a good **anthelmintic** herb and it can be useful to add this to the mares daily feed. It will cause a "tainted" taste to the milk but can only be of benefit.

All cases of scouring in a foal should be taken seriously. Where this condition continues it is important to seek veterinary treatment because the foal will quickly **dehydrate** with the loss of bodily fluids. Veterinary treatment will usually include prescription **anthelmentics**.

Externally the foal should be gently cleaned and dried. Warm water with a little salt added can be used and a good protective cream of **Tea Tree** can be applied to help heal and to act as a barrier against further infection.

Slippery Elm is another useful herb that can be fed to the foal. It should be mixed with a little of the mares milk and made into a paste. This can be syringed into the foals mouth up to four times a day.

MASTITIS

This condition is more common in cows where some believe the automatic milking machines can contribute. Normally with mares they are suckled naturally by the foal and it is certainly true to say that mastitis is unusual in a mare. Orthodox treatment involves **antibiotics** often syringed into the teat. This can be a painful condition for the mare and prevention is better than cure. It is reputed that **Cider Apple Vinegar** not only helps prevent mastitis but also improves the quality of the milk in the nursing mare.

In order to reduce the likelihood of infection, which often begins after a foal has been weaned and the milk is no longer being suckled, you can start feeding **Cider Apple Vinegar** at the rate of 25 mls a day as soon as the mare has a foal through until the foal has been weaned and she has "dried up".

MILK PRODUCTION

If a mare has a good balanced diet and plenty of spring grass she will usually produce an ample supply of milk for her foal. Some foodstuff can be particularly helpful such as **Alfalfa** and fresh green vegetables. Carrots are also good for the **lactating** mare as well as a number of herbs. The best known herb for stimulating milk production is **Fenugreek.** Others that can be used for this purpose are **Nettles, Aniseed** and **Fennel**.

To help to stop milk production after weaning you can feed **Mint** at the rate of 50 gms per day.

FERTILITY

The **fertility** in horses can be a matter of high finance, where a good pedigree classic winner promises to have a long and successful stud career. Whilst a mare can have only one foal each year it is normal for a top stallion to cover between 40 and 60 mares each year. It is simply because of the high sums of money involved that it has now become common practice to "manage" the covering of mares to maximise the chances of a successful full term **pregnancy**.

In their natural environment a stallion would run wild with his band of mares who would deter him from making amorous advances until they were in **oestrus** and ready to conceive. However, just because a mare is receptive to a stallion it does not follow that a conception will result. A stallion may be carrying an infectious venereal disease that he may pass from mare to mare. Also the greater the number of times a mare is covered the more likely she is to contract an infection that can prevent a conception. It is therefore normal at a professional stud for swabs to be taken from both the stallion and mare to ensure they are not carrying infection before covering takes place.

By ensuring that both the stallion and mare are free of disease and that the mare is covered at the correct time and as few times as possible, you are off to a reasonable start. However, there are a number of other factors that can effect the fertility in horses. Very occasionally a stallion may be found to be **infertile**. In such cases a laboratory examination of the semen will usually identify an abnormality which sometimes is not treatable with orthodox medicine. There are herbs that have a reputation of helping this problem such as **Damiana** and **Saw Palmetto** but it is difficult to separate the folk law from reality. Certainly these are worth trying if all else fails.

Although the Jockey Club of Great Britain and many other governing bodies require a natural covering to take place to register the progeny, it is now more and more common for **artificial insemination (A.I.)** to be used. This has the advantage that the semen is reliable, the risk of infection minimised, the mare is fully examined and the timing of insemination can be to suit the correct stage of the **oestrus cycle** in the mare. Another great advantage of this method is that **A.I.** can take place at the home of the mare. Often travelling a mare to a public stud for the services of a stallion can bring about its own problems where the mare can become **nervous** or **over-excitable**. Experienced mares may think they are travelling to compete again and get "wound-up" in the horse box. Also when a mare travels with a foal at foot there is always the possibility of injury to the foal.

Although mares generally tend to have different problems relating to their reproductive organs, the same herbs that are used for fertility in stallions may be helpful. The rate of conception begins to reduce rapidly as a mare gets older, and at the age of 15 years the likelihood of a **pregnancy** is less than 50%. When mares have had a number of foals this results in wear and tear to the **uterus** which in turn restricts the mares ability to maintain a **pregnancy**. The scarred walls of the **uterus** reduce the available area for a **foetus** to obtain nourishment. Some herbs have uterine tonic qualities and it is well worth considering feeding **Chaste Tree** and **Fenugreek** combined with **Echinacea** to help tone the **uterus** and build up the **immune system**.

RIG, FALSE RIG

Often when people talk about the behaviour in a male horse they may question if he is a rig. This term is used to describe a male horse where one of the testis fails to pass from the abdomen through the opening of the scrotum. This process usually takes place in the last months of gestation. Although sometimes where a testis has passed out of the abdomen but failed to descend into the scrotum, it may do so as the horse matures from the age of 2-3.

Any testis that does not reach the scrotum will not produce sperm. However, they will produce hormones resulting in stallion behaviour. It is believed that such a rig can be as a result of a genetic defect and therefore should not be used for breeding.

A false rig is where a male has been completely castrated but still displays masculine behaviour – anything from rounding up mares through to fully covering a mare in season. Where such behaviour is demonstrated blood tests can determine whether this is a rig or a false rig. Once it is confirmed that a horse that displays this type of behaviour has been fully castrated, then clearly it is a **behavioural problem** that needs careful management.

A herb that has been of benefit in such cases is **Chaste Tree** (**Agnus Castus**). This herb is more commonly used for regularising female **hormones** but as its other name **Monks Pepper** suggests, it is regarded as an antiaphrodisiac.

BEHAVIOUR

Behaviour	204
Over Excitable, Nervousness, Anxiety	205
Head Shaking	207
Stable vices	208
Weaving	208
Crib biting	208
Wind sucking	209

BEHAVIOUR

In dealing with behavioural problems it is necessary to have as much knowledge of the horse as possible. Bad behaviour can be the result of either psychological or physical problems and like most things with horses, good management will often help prevent and recognise the cause of a problem very early on.

Unfortunately some horses are labelled as "problem horses" and go through a series of hands, being passed on from one to the other – often making the situation worse. Too often young horses are started in life by inexperienced or unsympathetic hands, who do not recognise problems as they develop.

Where a problem in a horse is one that has recently occurred it is usually easier to find possible reasons. Apparent bad behaviour can be as a result of trying to avoid **pain**, and an unsound horse, or one whose saddle or bridle hurts, will naturally be reluctant to move in a way that increases the discomfort. By identifying the cause and removing the **pain**, progress is almost guaranteed.

In cases where problems may be related to discomfort or **pain** a veterinary surgeon can usually help in identifying the area concerned. Many causes are fundamental and a close examination of the behaviour change will usually give the clues. For example, a horse may throw its head about or behave unruly with a bad fitting bit, or one that puts pressure on a sore part of its mouth.

Where the problem is physical there are usually ways of helping with herbs – once you know what the problem is.

Psychological problems are not always easy to discover and often take a lot of understanding. For example, a horse that shies may have a genuine fear for a particular obstacle due to some previous bad experience.

Sometimes a horse can demonstrate **aggressive behaviour** towards other horses for no apparent reason. This can be as a result of being taken away or losing a close companion, or from some other change in the social circle of the horse. Horses also vary throughout the year through **hormonal changes** particularly mares during the spring and summer time when they often demonstrate both aggressive and friendly behaviour as they progress through the **oestrus cycle**. Likewise an entire horse or even a gelding can have very similar behavioural patterns particularly when being kept in close proximity to a mare or filly (see **Rig/False Rig**).

Where the behaviour is due to a **hormonal change** there are ways of helping this with herbs that have hormonal normalising and **sedative** type qualities. Often a combination of these can be very helpful, not only for regulating the **oestrus cycle** for breeding, but also in controlling **PMT (PMS)** and other hormonal related behaviour.

There are of course the common problems that are known as **stable vices**, such as **windsucking, crib biting, weaving** or box walking. A number of herbs can be helpful and they are dealt with under their own headings elsewhere.

EXCITABILITY, NERVOUSNESS, ANXIOUSNESS

Over excited, volatile, highly strung, anxious, apprehensive or worried behaviour in a horse is not always a demonstration of bad behaviour. A great number of factors can cause a horse to be anxious or have an overexcited or nervous reaction and it is important to try to understand the problem. **Calming** herbs are probably the biggest used of all and many can be effective in helping a horse to relax. However, if you can identify the cause of the problem it is much easier to deal with. In some cases **calming** herbs may not be the best approach and a good knowledge of your horses background and behavioural patterns will almost certainly help. Sometimes a horse is uneasy because of a previous bad experience. Occasionally an inexperienced rider or handler has brought about, or made worse, a problem because of their lack of understanding causing the horse to become stressed and worried.

In establishing the cause of irregular behaviour one needs to consider if the cause is **pain** related or through a lack of experience or **fear**.

Horses are by nature very insecure and it is natural that when asked to do something new, or repeat something that was not a good experience, there may be some hesitation. A horse that is overfed for the amount of exercise undertaken, may be more lively than their handlers wish sometimes causing it to buck just for the fun of it. Bucking may also be because of bad fitting tack or a back problem (see **McTimoney Chiropractic**). When a horse rears up it is usually to avoid something, possibly painful fitting headgear or as a demonstration of a reluctance to go forward due to some fear or previous experience. All of these are factors that can give the impression of an over excitable, nervous or reluctant horse.

If it is established that there is a need to relax the horse there are a number of herbs that are suitable. **Chamomile, Hops** and **Vervain** are well used whilst **Valerian** is a particularly effective **sedative** herb.

When teaching a horse new things herbs can help the pupil to have a more relaxed approach to learning. However, they are not a substitute for a bad teacher!

A question we are often asked is if relaxing herbs will adversely affect the horse's competition performance. The answer is that if the correct herbs are fed in reasonable quantities it is likely to improve the performance by reducing the amount of wasted nervous energy before the event, thus helping the horse to focus its effort to the task in hand.

It usually takes a week or so for herbs to get into the system so if you need to help a horse to relax before the big occasion you should start feeding at least a week beforehand.

Some horses come back from competitions still 'buzzing' and they are unable to relax or eat properly. In these cases it is necessary to relax the **digestive system** and a good way of doing this is to use an **infusion** of **Chamomile**. This can be fed in a syringe if necessary. Once the horse begins to eat, herbs can be added to the food.

HEAD SHAKING

The causes of head shaking are numerous and it is often difficult to establish the exact reason why a horse demonstrates this behaviour. Because this condition occurs more often in summer months it is often regarded as an allergic reaction to environmental factors, such as **pollen** or a sensitivity to sunlight.

The severity of head shaking varies, not only according to the sensitivity of the horse to environmental or other causes such as **mites** in the ears, but also to other factors that promote this behaviour. An unseen **tumour** or **growth** can cause irritation and obstruction to the **respiratory system**. Teeth and mouth problems as a result of infection or poor fitting tack are other reasons that have been known to cause head shaking.

Sometimes a horse may rub its nose indicating irritation of the nasal passage. In other cases the head shaking may only be apparent when a horse is being ridden, which is indicative of poor fitting tack, a reluctance to proceed through lameness or an inexperienced or unsympathetic rider.

In all cases it is necessary to look for the clues. Does it only occur in summer months? Is it worse when a horse is outside? Is it only apparent when the horse is ridden? If you can identify the cause you can normally deal with the problem.

STABLE VICES
The following section deals with common problems that are generally referred to as stable vices. In practice these can also relate to horses that are in the paddock.

WEAVING
Weaving is an annoying habit. A weaver will move its head from side to side in a rocking motion as it shifts weight from one front foot to the other. Occasionally this can be due to **pain** in the feet, but more often it is caused by bored or **anxious** behaviour. A normally relaxed horse may start weaving when it is close to feeding time or when attention is being sought.

Most horses will weave over the stable door looking out, and the simple installation of a "weave grill" will prevent this. However, more extreme weavers will do so in the middle of a stable, or field. In the stable a hanging ball or old tyre sometimes helps but outside it is more difficult.

Horses will copy this habit so it is important to reduce weaving where possible. Some **calming** herbs can reduce the incidence of weaving.

CRIB BITING
Crib biters will chew on stable doors, fences and other surfaces. Sometimes horses only crib bite when stabled, sometimes when turned out, or both. This habit can start due to some **vitamin** or **mineral** deficiency but it can also be a bad habit learned from another horse. A horse can also **crib bite** through **boredom** or to gain attention. For example, a horse that has grazed happily all day may start to crib bite on the fence when it is time to come in for feeding.

Firstly you should ensure that a horse has a good balanced diet to include the necessary **vitamins** and **minerals**. Prevention is better than cure therefore where possible remove or protect vulnerable surfaces. Where a horse chews on the lower door, connecting a top grill can cover the door edge so that it becomes inaccessible.

Boredom can play its part, particularly where a horse is edgy, or **highly strung** and is stabled for many hours. This is quite common in racing stables. First try to find the cause and the things that help. Some horses benefit from having a companion with them such as a goat, sheep or even a rabbit, whilst others find a ball or a car tyre hanging in the stable keeps them amused.

If management alone is not enough then it may be that some relaxing herbs will help. Gentle **sedatives** such as **Chamomile** can be effective and in more extreme cases **Valerian** may be used. The best approach may be a **calming** combination of herbs that complement each other.

WINDSUCKING

In most cases horses that windsuck also **crib bite**. Windsucking is almost a progression from **crib biting**. Windsucking is an unpleasant vice where a horse arches its neck and sucks in air with what sounds like a grunting noise. This is a vice other horses will copy and it is most important that you keep a windsucker out of sight and sound from other horses where possible. Having said that it is not always apparent why a horse sometimes starts to windsuck.

We once had a case where a young foal started to windsuck shortly after weaning. There was no history of windsucking from either parent and no other horse in the yard windsucked. Within three days the young foal in the next stable joined in the chorus of windsucking. We learned our lesson!

The fear is that windsucking can be instrumental in causing **colic** and it can affect **appetite**, condition and hence energy in a horse. Certainly in severe cases it can be difficult to get a horse to eat well if they are full of air!

Windsucking is fairly common in racehorses, and there are many examples of top class performers who were windsuckers. Also it does not follow that a windsucking mare will rear a foal with the same habit, although six months of teaching can rub off!

Management is the starting point in dealing with a windsucker. Like **crib biters** it is helpful to remove tempting edges and surfaces.

In order to windsuck a horse has to arch its neck. A way of preventing this is by applying a strap around the neck that is designed to limit this movement. Purpose made collars are available from a good saddler. In some cases an operation is carried out that involves removing a piece of muscle from the neck to restrict the movement. This seems somewhat barbaric. We have known of cases where it has worked and others where it lasted only for a limited time.

Sometimes moving a horse to a completely different stable can stop it **windsucking** for more than a week and changing stables on a regular basis to keep things interesting can be helpful. However, this does not always work and the stress of a change in some cases will make things worse.

Sedative and **relaxing** herbs can be helpful as part of an overall management programme. It is unusual to cure windsucking but it is possible to control or reduce it.

BOX REST

Box rest is sometimes unavoidable. Where a horse has an injury that requires reduced movement to heal, it is standard practice for a veterinary surgeon to order box rest. Indeed, even where a problem has not been fully diagnosed the first course of action may be box rest, hence giving nature the opportunity of healing and repairing.

Herbs can make a useful contribution to the well being of a horse who requires box rest in various ways. They can help with the condition itself – relieving **pain**, reducing swelling and quickening the healing process depending on the diagnosis and veterinary advice.

When a horse is suddenly confined to the stable after being used to daily exercise or turnout, this brings about a big change in the routine. Particular attention needs to be paid to diet and bedding. A reduction in concentrated feed is necessary and in some cases the veterinary surgeon may suggest feeding good quality hay only, especially if there has been some **digestive problem**. It is important to monitor droppings and, if anything, they need to be on the soft side. If a horse is being given **antibiotics** or treatment for **colic** or has a digestive upset they may be too soft. If the droppings are on the firm side or even normal the addition of sunflower oil or **laxative** herbs to the diet may be helpful.

Bedding should be kept clean and dry to avoid foot infection. There is the likelihood of the horse eating the bedding through reduced diet and **boredom** and this must be avoided because it can lead to **colic**. Where there is any risk of this, the bedding should be changed for shavings or paper.

A good clean water supply should be available continuously. It is helpful to monitor intake of water. Therefore, buckets are better than an automatic supply for this purpose. Observe the passing of urine and droppings by carefully checking the bedding. Where there is a shortfall in either, the veterinary surgeon should be made aware. When a horse "stands in" it may have **filled legs** as a result of inactivity. If necessary **diuretic** herbs can help to increase the flow of urine.

Another problem with confining a horse is that it can become overactive, **excitable** or **anxious** at being on its own when it is separated from its friends. **Sedative** and relaxing herbs can play a useful part in the early stages of adjusting to the new situation and if necessary can be an aid to keeping the horse calm when it has to be introduced to gradual exercise.

EYE PROBLEMS

Occasionally a foreign object such as a thorn or a husk from grain may cause swelling or weeping of the eye. If early action is taken it is often possible to remove this by gently bathing the eye with warm water.

Eyes will sometimes weep due to an **allergic reaction** to environmental factors such as **pollen,** which may give **hay fever** type symptoms.

A herb that is particularly good for eye problems such as **conjunctivitis** and **keratitis** is **Eyebright**. This can be made into a **decoction** and when it cools down should be strained to remove all particles of the herb before using as an eye wash.

The problem with ailments of the eye is that the natural reaction is for the eyelid to close and often the resultant swelling makes treatment difficult. Where necessary a veterinary surgeon can administer a local anaesthetic and in all but the simplest of cases veterinary assistance should be sought.

USEFUL ADDRESSES

Wendals Herbs Ltd
The Chase, Chalk Road, Walpole St. Peter, Wisbech, Cambs. PE14 7PN.
Telephone: 01945 780880
www.wendals.com
Fax: 01945 780044
U.S. Freephone: 1 800 981 0320
Specialist producers of quality herbal products for horses.

Equi-Ternatives
96 CR 536, Bushnell, Florida. 33513. U.S.A
Telephone: 352 569 0410
Fax: 352 569 0406
U.S distributors of Wendals Herbs products.

Toklat Originals Inc.
PO Box 488, Lake Oswego, Oregon. 97034. U.S.A
Telephone: 503 636 6212
Fax: 503 636 6296
U.S national distributors of Wendals Herbs products.

British Association of Holistic Nutrition & Medicine
Borough Court, Hartley Witney, Basingstoke, Hants. RG27 8JA.
Telephone: 01252 843282
Advisors and licencing body for Holistic products.

British Horse Society
Stoneleigh Deer Park, Kenilworth, Warwickshire. CV8 2XZ.
Telephone: 01926 707700
www.bhs.org.uk
Fax: 01926 707800

USEFUL ADDRESSES

International League for the Protection of Horses
Anne Colvin House, Snetterton, Norwich, Norfolk. NR16 2LR.
Telephone: 01953 498682
www.ilph.org   Fax: 01953 498373

Bach Flower Essences
Foundation, The Bach Centre, Mount Vernon, Bakers Lane, Sotwell, Oxon. OX10 0PZ.
Telephone: 01491 834678
www.bachflower.com   Fax: 01491 825022

McTimoney Chiropractic College
The Clock House, 22-26 Ock Street, Abingdon, Oxford. OX14 5SH.
Telephone: 01235 523336
Fax: 01235 523576

Chiropractic@mctimoney-college.ac.uk

GLOSSARY

A.I.	Artificial Insemination
Bile	Secreted by the liver to aid the digestion of fats.
Bute	Abbreviated name for Phenylbutazone
Carbohydrates	Energy providing nutrients.
Cast	When a horse has rolled into a position (usually upside down, against a wall) where it is unable to extend its front legs on the floor to get up.
Choke	An obstruction of the oesophagus (gullet).
Chronic	Long suffering.
Cyst	A secreting closed cavity.
Electrolytes	The bodies natural salts: Sodium Chloride, Sodium, Bicarbonate, Potassium Chloride solution in the body.
Fat	A concentrated source of energy.
Foal heat	Oestrus period about ten days after foaling.
Fungal Infection	An infection caused by fungus, eg. Ringworm.
Gutteral pouch	Air sacs situated between the pharynx and the floor of the skull.
Intravenous	Into a vein.
Jaundice	A yellowness of the skin relating to the discharge of bile pigment from the liver.

GLOSSARY

Lactation — Secretion of milk from the udder.

Lame — Unsound.

Mucus — Lubricates the airways collecting dust and other particles sometimes discharging through the nostrils.

Ovary — Organ of the female reproductive system.

Ovulation — Follicle release from the ovary.

Pancreas — A gland which lies in the abdomen that aids the digestive system.

Phenylbutazone — A drug with analgesic and anti-inflammatory actions.

Photosensitization — The process that renders skin or other tissue abnormally sensitive to light.

Proteins — A combination of amino acids to maintain and develop healthy tissue.

Puss — Fluid product of inflammation.

Sutured — Surgically stitched.

Uterus — Cavity in the female that houses a developing foetus.

Virus — An infective agent not identifiable as bacterium.

Index

A brief background to herbs	11	Antiseptic	111
Abdominal pain	140	Antispasmodic	112
Abrasions	179	Anti-tumour	82
Abscesses	177	Antiviral	112
Achillea millefolium	104	Anxiousness	205
Acrid	109	Aperient	112
Aggressive behaviour	204	Aphrodisiac	112
Agnus castus	40	Apium graveolens	37
Agropyron repens	45	Appetiser	112
A.I.	Glossary	Appetite	139
Alfalfa	25	Arctium lappa	35
Allergic reaction (skin)	171	Arnica	28
Allergies (respiratory)	158	Arnica montana	28
Allium sativum	55	Aromatherapy	129
Aloe	26	Aromatic	112
Aloe barbadensis	26	Artemisia absinthium	103
Alterative	109	Arthritis	182
Althaea officinalis	71	Artificial insemination	Glossary
Anaemia	163	Ascarrids	147
Analgesic	109	Ascorbic acid	125
Angleberry	177	Asthma	158
Aniseed	27	Astringent	113
Anodyne	109	Azoturia	183
Anoestrus	194		
Anoplocephala perfoliata	150	Bach flower remedies	132
Antacid	109	Bacterial infections	157
Anthelmintic	109	BAHNM	14
Antibacterial	109	Balm	30
Antibiotic	110	Basil	32
Anticatarrhal	110	Behaviour	203
Antidepressant	110	Behavioural problems	204
Antifungal	110	Benign tumour	175
Antigalactagogue	110	Bile	Glossary
Antihistamine	110	Biotin	125
Antihypothyroid	110	Bitter	113
Anti-inflammatory	111	Bladder infection	167
Antilithic	111	Bladderwrack	33
Antimicrobial	111	Bleeding (EIPH)	156
Antipyretic	111	Blood	163
Antirheumatic	111	Bone marrow	163

- 219 -

Index

Bots	150	Compound fracture	190
Box rest	211	Conjunctivitis	212
Broken wind	158	Constipation	143
Bruised sole	188	COPD	158
Bruising	189	Copper	122
Buckwheat	34	Couch Grass	45
Burdock	35	Coughing	158
Bursting	156	Cracked heels	174
Bute	Glossary	Crataegus oxyacantha	60
		Crib biting	208
Cajeput	95	Cushings disease	165
Calciferol	126	Cyanocobalamin	124
Calcium	121	Cyst	175
Calendula officinalis	68	Cystitis	167
Calmative	113		
Calming	205	Damiana	48
Cancer	175	Dandelion	46
Carbohydrates	Glossary	Decoction	127
Cardiac tonic	113	Degenerative joint disease	182
Carminative	113	Dehydration	145
Celery	37	Demulcent	114
Chamomile	38	Dermatitis	174
Chaste Tree	40	Devils Claw	49
Chills	167	Diaphoretic	114
Chiropractic	133	Diarrhoea	144
Choke	Glossary	Dictyocaulus arnfieldi	149
Cholagogue	113	Digestive system	137
Choline	125	Dioestrus	194
Choosing herbal products	13	Diuretic	114
Chronic	Glossary	DJD	182
Chronic obstructive pulmonary disease	158		
Circulatory system	161	Echinacea	50
Cleavers	41	Echinacea angustifolia	50
Clivers	41	EHVI subtype 1	157
Coat	169	EIPH	156
Colic	140	Electrolytes	Glossary
Coltsfoot	42	Emmenagogue	114
Comfrey	44	Emollient	114
Common names	19	Enteritis	144

Index

Epistaxis	156	Garlic	55
Equine asthma	158	Gaseous colic	141
Equine hepevirus	157	Ginkgo	58
Equine Influenza	157	Ginkgo biloba	58
Equisetum arvense	63	Glands	163
Essence	128	Glandular problems	163
Euphrasia officinalis	52	Glycyrrhiza glabra	67
Excitability	205	Golden Rod	56
Exercise induced pulmonary haemorrhage	156	Goose grass	41
Expectorant	115	Grass sickness	143
Eye problems	212	Greasy heels	174
Eyebright	52	Green ginger	103
		Growths	175
False Rig	201	Guttural pouch	Glossary
Fat	Glossary		
Fat soluble	125	Haemostatic	115
Fear	205	Hamamelis virginiana	102
Febrifuge	115	Harpagophytum procumbens	49
Feeding guide	17	Hawthorn	60
Feeding guidelines	15	Hay fever	158
Fennel	53	Head shaking	207
Fenugreek	54	Heaves	158
Fertility	199	Hepatic	115
Filled legs	172	Herb actions	109
Filpendula ulmaria	72	Highly strung	205
Flies	173	Hives	172
Foal scour	197	Homeopathy	131
Foaling	196	Hoof	187
Foaling heat	Glossary	Hops	59
Foeniculum vulgare	53	Horehound	62
Folic acid	124	Hormonal changes	194
Founders	186	Hormonal disorders	163
Fracture	190	Hormonal system	163
Fragaria vesca	94	Hormones	163
Fucus vesiculosis	33	Horsetail	63
Fungal infection	Glossary	Humulus lupulus	59
		Hyperactivity	205
Galactogogue	115	Hypericum perforatum	92
Galium aparine	41	Hyperthyroidism	164

Index

Hypnotic	115	Lymph glands	164
Hypothroidism	164	Lymphangitis	164
		Lymphatic system	164
Immune system	166		
Immuno-stimulant	115	Magnesium	121
Impactive colic	141	Malignant tumour	175
Infertile	200	Manganese	122
Inflammation	191	Marigold	68
Infusion	127	Marjoram	70
Insect bites	173	Marrubium vulgare	62
Intravenous	Glossary	Marshmallow	71
Iodine	123	Mastitis	198
Iron	122	Materia Medica	23
		Matricaria chamomilla	38
Jaundice	Glossary	McTimoney Chiropractic	133
		Meadowsweet	72
Kelp	33	Medicago sativa	25
Keratitis	212	Melaleuca leucadendron	95
Kidney	167	Melanomas	176
Kidney infections	167	Melissa officinalis	30
Knitbone	44	Mentha piperita	75
		Midges	171
Lactating	Glossary	Milk production	199
Lactoflavin	124	Milk Thistle	74
Lameness	Glossary	Minerals	121
Laminitis	186	Mint	75
Large strongyles	148	Monks Pepper	40
Latin names	21	Mucilage	116
Lavandula officinalis	64	Mucus	Glossary
Lavender	64	Mud fever	174
Laxative	116	Muscle sprains	184
Lemon Balm	30	Muscular & Skeletal system	181
Lice	173		
Ligament strain or damage	185	Nasal discharge	155
Lime Tree	66	Nasal food discharge	156
Liquorice	67	Nasal haemorraging	156
Liver	146	Navicular syndrome	187
Liver problems	146	Nervine	116
Lucerne	25	Nervousness	205
Lungworm	149	Nettle	76

Index

Nettle rash	172	Polygonum fogopyrum	34
Niacin	124	Potassium	121
Nits	173	Poultice	128
		Powder	128
Ocimum basilicum	32	Pregnancy	195
Oedema	179	Protein	Glossary
Oestrus	194	Psyllium	80
Oestrus cycle	194	Purple Clover	82
Ointment	128	Pus	Glossary
Origanum vulgare	70		
Other herbal preparations	127	Rain scald	174
Ovary	Glossary	Raspberry	81
Over excitable	205	Red cells	163
Overactive Thyroid	164	Red Clover	82
Ovulation	Glossary	Red Poppy	83
Oxyuris equi	149	Red sage	88
		Redworm	148
Pain relief	191	Relaxant	116
Pancreas	Glossary	Relaxing herbs	206
Papaver rhoeas	83	Reproductive system	193
Parascaris equorum	148	Respiratory system	153
Parasitic infestation	147	Restorative	116
Parsley	78	Retinol	125
Parturient	116	Rheumatism	182
Pectoral	116	Rhinopnumonitis	157
Peppermint	75	Riboflavin	124
Periwinkle	79	Rig	201
Petroselinum crispum	78	Ringworm	172
Phenylbutazone	Glossary	Rosa canina	84
Phosphorus	121	Rosehips	84
Photosensitization	Glossary	Rosemary	86
Pigmentation	178	Rosmarinus officinalis	86
Pimpinella anisum	27	Round worm	148
Pinworms	149	Rubefacient	117
Pituitary gland	164	Rubus idaeus	81
Plantago psyllium	80		
Plasma	163	Sage	88
Pleurisy	160	Salix alba	101
PMT/PMS	194	Salvia officinalis	88
Pneumonia	159	Sand colic	142

- 223 -

Index

Sarcoids	177	Tapeworm	150
Saw Palmetto	90	Taraxacum officinale	46
Scouring	197	Tea Tree	95
Scratches	174	Tendon and ligament damage	185
Seatworm	149	Thiamin	124
Seaweed	33	Threadworm	147
Sedative	117	Thrush	189
Selenium	123	Thyme	96
Serenoa serrulata	90	Thymus vulgaris	96
Set fast	183	Thyroid gland	164
Silyburn marianum	74	Tics	173
Simple fracture	190	Tilia europaea	66
Sinus discharge	155	Tincture	128
Skin	169	Tissue healing	44
Skin allergies	171	Tocopherol	126
Skin irritations	171	Tonic	118
Slippery Elm	91	Trace elements	122
Small strongyles	147	Trefoil	82
Sodium	122	Trichonema species	148
Solidago virgaurea	56	Trifolium pratense	82
Sore feet	188	Trigonella foenum - graecum	54
Spasmodic colic	140	Tumour	175
Spasmolytic	117	Turnera aphrodisiaca	48
Spleen	163	Tussilago farfara	42
Spotted alder	102	Twisted gut	142
St Johns Wort	92	Tying up	183
Stable cough	158		
Stable vices	208	Ulmus fulva	91
Stimulant	117	Underactive thyroid	164
Stomachic	117	Urinary system	167
Strangles	177	Urine infections	167
Strawberry	94	Urtica dioica	76
Streptococcus equi infection	177	Uterus	Glossary
Strongyloides western	147		
Strongylus vulgaris	148	Valerian	98
Sutured	Glossary	Valeriana officinalis	98
Sweating	146	Verbena officinalis	100
Sweet itch	171	Vermifuge	118
Symphytum officinale	44	Vervain	100

Index

Vinca major	79
Viral infections	157
Virus	Glossary
Vitamin A	125
Vitamin B1	124
Vitamin B12	124
Vitamin B2	124
Vitamin B3	124
Vitamin C	125
Vitamin D	126
Vitamin E	126
Vitamin K	126
Vitamins & minerals	119
Vulnerary	118
Warts	176
Water soluble vitamins	124
Weaving	208
Weight loss	145
Wet the bed	46
White cells	163
White Horehound	62
White tea tree	95
White Willow	101
Willow	101
Windsucking	209
Winterbloom	102
Witch Hazel	102
Worming	150
Worms	147
Wormwood	103
Wounds	178
Yarrow	104
Zinc	122

NOTES